Psychological Approaches to Cancer Care

About the Authors

Teresa L. Deshields, PhD, ABPP, is the Director of Supportive Oncology at Rush University Cancer Center and a professor in the Departments of Medicine, and Psychiatry and Behavioral Sciences at Rush University Medical Center in Chicago. She is a clinical health psychologist, and her clinical practice is devoted to treating cancer patients and their family members, throughout the cancer continuum. Her research is focused on issues related to symptom burden and quality of life in cancer patients and survivors.

Jonathan L. Kaplan, MD, is an assistant professor in the Departments of Psychiatry and Behavioral Sciences and Medicine at Rush University Medical Center. He is the psychiatrist for the Rush University Cancer Center and a consultation–liaison psychiatrist at Rush University Medical Center. He specializes in the psychiatric treatment of medically complex patients including patients with cancer. His research interests include psycho-oncology and collaborative care psychiatry.

Lauren Z. Rynar, PhD, is an assistant professor in the Department of Psychiatry and Behavioral Sciences and a clinician in the supportive oncology program at the Rush University Cancer Center. She specializes in the psychological care of cancer patients, survivors, and caregivers. Her research interests include quality of life, coping styles, cancer-related distress, and models of supportive care delivery among cancer patients.

Advances in Psychotherapy – Evidence-Based Practice

Series Editor
Danny Wedding, PhD, MPH, Professor Emeritus, University of Missouri–Saint Louis, MO

Associate Editors
Jonathan S. Comer, PhD, Professor of Psychology and Psychiatry, Director of Mental Health Interventions and Technology (MINT) Program, Center for Children and Families, Florida International University, Miami, FL
J. Kim Penberthy, PhD, ABPP, Professor of Psychiatry & Neurobehavioral Sciences, University of Virginia, Charlottesville, VA
Kenneth E. Freedland, PhD, Professor of Psychiatry and Psychology, Washington University School of Medicine, St. Louis, MO
Linda C. Sobell, PhD, ABPP, Professor, Center for Psychological Studies, Nova Southeastern University, Ft. Lauderdale, FL

The basic objective of this series is to provide therapists with practical, evidence-based treatment guidance for the most common disorders seen in clinical practice – and to do so in a reader-friendly manner. Each book in the series is both a compact "how-to" reference on a particular disorder for use by professional clinicians in their daily work and an ideal educational resource for students as well as for practice-oriented continuing education.

The most important feature of the books is that they are practical and easy to use: All are structured similarly and all provide a compact and easy-to-follow guide to all aspects that are relevant in real-life practice. Tables, boxed clinical "pearls," marginal notes, and summary boxes assist orientation, while checklists provide tools for use in daily practice.

Continuing Education Credits

Psychologists and other healthcare providers may earn five continuing education credits for reading the books in the *Advances in Psychotherapy* series and taking a multiple-choice exam. This continuing education program is a partnership of Hogrefe Publishing and the National Register of Health Service Psychologists. Details are available at https://www.hogrefe.com/us/cenatreg

The National Register of Health Service Psychologists is approved by the American Psychological Association to sponsor continuing education for psychologists. The National Register maintains responsibility for this program and its content.

Advances in Psychotherapy – Evidence-Based Practice, Volume 46

Psychological Approaches to Cancer Care

Teresa L. Deshields
Jonathan L. Kaplan
Lauren Z. Rynar

Rush University Medical Center, Chicago, IL

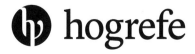

Library of Congress of Congress Cataloging in Publication information for the print version of this book is available via the Library of Congress Marc Database under the Library of Congress Control Number 2022936270

Library and Archives Canada Cataloguing in Publication

Title: Psychological approaches to cancer care / Teresa L. Deshields, Jonathan L. Kaplan, Lauren Z. Rynar.
Names: Deshields, Teresa L., author. | Kaplan, Jonathan L., author. | Rynar, Lauren Z., author.
Series: Advances in psychotherapy--evidence-based practice ; v. 46.
Description: Series statement: Advances in psychotherapy--evidence-based practice ; volume 46 |
  Includes bibliographical references and index.
Identifiers: Canadiana (print) 20220219532 | Canadiana (ebook) 20220219567 | ISBN 9780889375116
  (softcover) | ISBN 9781616765118 (PDF) | ISBN 9781613345115 (EPUB)
Subjects: LCSH: Cancer—Psychological aspects. | LCSH: Cancer—Patients—Care. | LCSH: Cancer—Patients—
  Mental health.
Classification: LCC RC262 .D47 2022 | DDC 616.99/40019—dc23

PUBLISHING OFFICES

USA: Hogrefe Publishing Corporation, 44 Merrimac St., Suite 207, Newburyport, MA 01950
                    Phone 978 255 3700; E-mail customersupport@hogrefe.com

EUROPE: Hogrefe Publishing GmbH, Merkelstr. 3, 37085 Göttingen, Germany
                    Phone +49 551 99950 0, Fax +49 551 99950 111; E-mail publishing@hogrefe.com

SALES & DISTRIBUTION

USA: Hogrefe Publishing, Customer Services Department,
                    30 Amberwood Parkway, Ashland, OH 44805
                    Phone 800 228 3749, Fax 419 281 6883; E-mail customersupport@hogrefe.com

UK: Hogrefe Publishing, c/o Marston Book Services Ltd., 160 Eastern Ave.,
                    Milton Park, Abingdon, OX14 4SB
                    Phone +44 1235 465577, Fax +44 1235 465556; E-mail direct.orders@marston.co.uk

EUROPE: Hogrefe Publishing, Merkelstr. 3, 37085 Göttingen, Germany
                    Phone +49 551 99950 0, Fax +49 551 99950 111; E-mail publishing@hogrefe.com

OTHER OFFICES

CANADA: Hogrefe Publishing Corporation, 82 Laird Drive, East York, Ontario M4G 3V1

SWITZERLAND: Hogrefe Publishing, Länggass-Strasse 76, 3012 Bern

ISBN 978-0-88937-511-6 (print) • ISBN 978-1-61676-511-8 (PDF) • ISBN 978-1-61334-511-5 (EPUB)
https://doi.org/10.1027/00511-000

Contents

1   **Description** 1
1.1   Common Psychiatric Diagnoses in the Context of Cancer 2
1.1.1   Major Depression 2
1.1.2   Adjustment Disorder 2
1.1.3   Anxiety Disorders 2
1.2   Other Psychiatric/Psychological Issues 3
1.2.1   Severe Mental Illness and Cancer 3
1.2.2   Distress 3
1.2.3   Fear of Recurrence 3
1.3   Epidemiology 4
1.4   Course and Prognosis 4
1.4.1   Vulnerable Periods 4
1.4.2   Trajectories of Psychological Distress 5
1.4.3   Posttraumatic Growth 5
1.4.4   Survivorship 6
1.5   Differential Diagnosis 6
1.6   Comorbidities 6
1.7   Diagnostic Procedures and Documentation 7
1.7.1   Distress Screening 7
1.7.2   Symptom Assessment 7
1.7.3   Depression Assessment 8
1.7.4   Anxiety Assessment 8
1.7.5   Quality of Life (QoL) 8

2   **Theories and Models** 10
2.1   Biopsychosocial Model of Cancer 10
2.2   Models of Cancer-Related Distress 13
2.2.1   Cancer-Related Distress as an Adjustment Disorder 13
2.2.2   Self-Regulatory Model of Illness Behavior 14
2.2.3   Stressful Life Events and the Impact of Coping Style on
        Cancer-Related Distress 15

3   **Diagnosis and Treatment Indications** 17
3.1   Distress in Cancer 17
3.2   Adjustment Disorders 18
3.3   Major Depressive Disorder 20
3.4   Anxiety Disorders 21
3.4.1   Generalized Anxiety Disorder (GAD) 21
3.4.2   Panic Disorder 23
3.4.3   Specific Phobias 24
3.5   Trauma-Related Disorders 24
3.5.1   Acute Stress Disorder 24
3.5.2   Posttraumatic Stress Disorder 25
3.6   Cognitive Dysfunction Secondary to Cancer Treatment 26

3.7	Substance Use Disorders (SUD)	28
3.8	Vulnerable Populations	30
4	**Treatment**	32
4.1	Methods of Treatment	33
4.1.1	Psychotherapy	33
4.1.2	Groups and Other Approaches	37
4.1.3	Medications	38
4.1.4	Future Directions	50
4.2	Effectiveness of Treatments	53
4.2.1	Psychosocial Interventions	53
4.2.2	Psychotropic Medications	53
4.3	Challenges in Delivering Treatment	55
4.3.1	Access Concerns for Treatment	55
4.3.2	Presence of Family/Caretakers	56
4.3.3	High Burden of Disease	57
4.3.4	The Therapist's Personal Experience With Cancer	57
4.3.5	Burnout/Compassion Fatigue	57
4.3.6	End-of-Life Care	58
4.4	Multicultural Issues	58
4.4.1	Diversity Issues	58
4.4.2	Religious Beliefs and Decision-Making About Treatment	59
5	**Case Vignettes**	60
5.1	Case Vignette 1: Ms. R.	60
5.2	Case Vignette 2: Mr. J.	63
6	**Further Reading**	66
7	**References**	67
8	**Appendix: Tools and Resources**	78

1

Description

Many people think of cancer as a single disease, with multiple possible sites of impact. In truth, cancer is a family of disorders with varying degrees of severity, prognosis, life disruption, impact on appearance, etc. There are other common misunderstandings, or myths, about cancer and its treatment. These are reviewed in Appendix 1. Treatment can be acute and time-limited, or it can be chronic and lifelong. The length of survivorship after a cancer diagnosis is widely variable, including some patients who will live with the disease and some who will be cured. Of course, the impact of cancer on any individual's mental health and quality of life is also greatly variable. There is also growing recognition of the impact of a cancer diagnosis on the family caregivers of the person with the diagnosis.

While cancer remains the second leading cause of death in the US, the death rate associated with cancer dropped every year between 1999 and 2019 (Centers for Disease Control and Prevention (CDC), 2021). This is generally attributed to decreases in cigarette smoking, increased utilization of cancer screening tests, and advances in cancer treatment. As death rates have dropped, there are increasing numbers of cancer survivors and longer periods of survivorship.

Although cancer rates are declining year by year, cancer is still the second leading cause of death in the United States

Psycho-oncology is a subspecialty in oncology, focused on the psychosocial impact of cancer on patients at all stages of the disease, on their families, as well as on individuals determined to be at increased risk for cancer. Psychosocial care in oncology is most typically provided by psychologists, social workers, nurses, and physicians, but it can also be provided by chaplains, patient navigators, and counselors (Deshields et al., 2013). For the psychosocial clinician, it can be difficult to learn the "language" of cancer care. Basic cancer terms are defined in Appendix 2.

Psycho-oncology is a subspecialty of oncology, focused on the psychosocial impact of cancer on patients and their families

While psycho-oncology clinicians often address psychiatric disorders, they also have occasion to provide care for those suffering from cancer with subclinical coping difficulties. Some appropriate targets for intervention may not rise to the level of a disorder, such as questions about how to communicate about the cancer diagnosis at work or with children, or dealing with hair loss, or concerns about sexuality after cancer treatment. We provide strategies that can be used in the context of clinical disorders or the context of coping challenges. Some clinicians may be working in settings where there is no concern about billing, but in those settings where billing is a concern, health and behavior codes may be appropriate for patients without a psychiatric diagnosis. Some patients may be willing to self-pay for psychosocial services.

1.1   Common Psychiatric Diagnoses in the Context of Cancer

1.1.1   Major Depression

The prevalence of major depression in the oncology population is estimated to be up to 24%

The prevalence of major depression in the oncology population is estimated to range up to 24% (Krebber et al., 2014). There can be overlap among the vegetative symptoms of depression (change in appetite, weight gain or loss, anergia, and change in sleep whether insomnia or excessive sleep) and symptoms of cancer or side effects of treatment. There can also be overlap among the cognitive/emotional symptoms of depression (feelings of guilt, concentration difficulties, thoughts of death) and reactions to cancer or to cancer treatment. Because anhedonia is one of the diagnostic criteria for depression and is not a side effect of cancer treatment, it may help the clinician to distinguish major depression from a general reaction to cancer.

1.1.2   Adjustment Disorder

Adjustment disorder may be present in up to 19% of patients with cancer

Adjustment Disorder may be present in up to 19% of patients in this population (van Beek et al., 2019). Adjustment Disorder is most commonly further defined by "with depression," "with anxiety," or "with mixed anxiety and depression." While Adjustment Disorder may be hard to distinguish from distress (described below), the diagnosis requires impairment in functioning.

1.1.3   Anxiety Disorders

The prevalence of anxiety disorders in patients with cancer is 11%

The prevalence of anxiety disorders in patients with cancer is estimated to be around 11% (Mehnert et al., 2014). Several types of anxiety disorders are more likely to be problematic in the cancer setting.

Generalized Anxiety Disorder (GAD)
GAD is characterized by persistent and pervasive worry. There is much to worry about in the cancer setting, including upcoming scans, the efficacy of treatment, the possibility of recurrence or progression of the disease, and the probability of death. Learning how to manage anxiety/worry is an important skill for those diagnosed with cancer and is addressed later.

Obsessive-Compulsive Disorder
In the cancer setting, obsessive concern about exposure to germs can become an issue, particularly for immunocompromised patients. Compulsive self-examination for the presence or progression of tumors can lead to irritation of relevant parts of the body, and the resulting swelling or tenderness can increase anxiety.

Phobia

Some phobias are particularly problematic in the cancer setting. A needle phobia can be very disruptive, especially for patients who require chemotherapy infusions, but it is also an issue because of the volume of routine blood draws required over the course of cancer care. Claustrophobia can be an issue during scans (particularly MRIs), but it can also be an issue if patients feel trapped by medical devices (during chemotherapy or radiation therapy) or in a hospital room.

1.2 Other Psychiatric/Psychological Issues

1.2.1 Severe Mental Illness and Cancer

Anyone can develop cancer, including those with pre-existing severe mental illness. Some literature suggests that this population is more vulnerable to worse cancer outcomes because of disparities in cancer screening and decreased likelihood of receiving appropriate cancer treatment (Grassi & Riba, 2020). Individuals with a psychiatric diagnosis are also screened for cancer less frequently than the general population (Solmi et al., 2020). Those with a psychiatric history are less likely to receive guideline-concordant cancer treatment and to receive timely treatment, resulting in worse medical outcomes (Kisely et al., 2013). Furthermore, cancer diagnosis and treatment have been associated with exacerbation of pre-existing psychiatric conditions (Hill et al., 2011).

1.2.2 Distress

Distress management has been advocated in cancer settings for many years but has been widely prevalent since 2015 when it became an accreditation standard for the American College of Surgeons Commission on Cancer (CoC; 2015). Distress is broadly defined by the National Comprehensive Cancer Network (NCCN) as a "multifactorial, unpleasant experience of a psychological, social, spiritual, and/or physical nature that may interfere with the ability to cope effectively with cancer, its physical symptoms, and its treatment" (NCCN, 2021, p. DIS-1). The prevalence of distress in cancer patients varies by type and stage of cancer, time since diagnosis, and sex, and ranges between 20% and 52% of cancer patients (Mehnert et al., 2018). Higher distress has been associated with increased utilization of medical resources, longer hospital stays, and poorer quality of life (QoL) (Götze et al., 2014; Nipp et al., 2017).

> **Distress screening became common when the COC made it an accreditation standard for cancer centers in 2015**

1.2.3 Fear of Recurrence

Fear of Cancer Recurrence (FCR) is defined as "fear, worry, or concern relating to the possibility that cancer will come back or progress" (Lebel et al., 2016, p. 3266). FCR is of clinical concern when the following characteristics are present: (1) high levels of preoccupation; (2) high levels of worry; (3) hypervigilance for symptoms/sensations suggesting recurrence; and (4) persistent worry, fear, or anxiety (Mutsaers et al., 2020). FCR is an issue in up to 87% of cancer survivors, and can be associated with psychological difficulties (Simard et al., 2013).

1.3   Epidemiology

Because the death rate associated with cancer is dropping, there is an increasing number of cancer survivors

The incidence of cancer is higher in men than women and slightly higher in whites than in other ethnicities (US Cancer Statistics Working Group, 2020). The incidence rate for all cancers combined for men in the US is 494.8 per 100,000, for women 419.3 per 100,000 (American Cancer Society [ACS], 2019). Cancer incidence increases with age, but the risk is also increased with smoking history, excessive body weight, alcohol consumption, and family history of cancer (ACS, 2019). As noted previously, from 1999 to 2019, the death rate from cancer decreased by 27%, reflecting improved treatment, reduced rates of smoking, and better cancer screening (CDC, 2021).

Psychosocial factors have also been associated with cancer and with adjustment to cancer. While death rates for cancer have been dropping overall, socioeconomic disparities in survival have grown over this same period (Siegel et al., 2019). Furthermore, the LGBTQ population is at greater risk for poor cancer outcomes (Quinn et al., 2015). Finally, patients with pre-existing mental illness have a poorer cancer-specific prognosis and survival rate (Kisely et al., 2013).

1.4   Course and Prognosis

Certain individuals are at greater risk than the general population for experiencing psychological distress in association with a cancer diagnosis. Not surprisingly, those with a history of a psychiatric disorder, substance use disorder (SUD), attempted suicide, trauma, or abuse are vulnerable to increased emotional difficulties in the context of cancer (NCCN, 2021). A variety of social issues also make psychological distress more likely in general, including family conflict, inadequate social support, financial difficulties, and lack of stable housing. Patients with certain types of cancer, including head and neck cancer and pancreatic cancer, are at greater risk for depression (Rohde et al., 2018). In cancer patients, younger age is associated with greater distress (Sansom-Daly & Wakefield, 2013). Furthermore, in cancer patients, symptom burden is negatively correlated with QoL (Deshields et al., 2014).

1.4.1   Vulnerable Periods

While the medical workup around a cancer diagnosis can be complicated and distressing, the course of treatment can be extended over months or years, with the latter more common in metastatic (stage 4) disease. Some patients never "finish" their treatment, and their cancer experience may be more comparable to other chronic illnesses, such as diabetes (more continuous) or asthma (more episodic). Certain timepoints across the cancer trajectory have been associated with increased risk of psychological difficulties (NCCN, 2021). Risk is highest at the time of cancer diagnosis (including the period of medical workup), disease progression or recurrence, upon anticipation of a new treatment, during hospitalization, and around the end-of-life. Interestingly, the conclusion of treatment can be a time of increased vulnerability to distress (NCCN, 2021). Some patients have acute episodes of anxiety in anticipation of surveillance imaging, a phenomenon labeled "scan-xiety" (Bauml et al., 2016).

Timepoints associated with increased psychological distress: cancer work-up/diagnosis, start of new treatment, surveillance scans, end of treatment, progression or recurrence of disease, and end-of-life

1.4.2   Trajectories of Psychological Distress

Some researchers have examined the trajectories of distress in cancer patients. Bonanno (2004) proposed a widely used model of trajectories of response to trauma. Deshields et al. (2006) examined Bonanno's trajectories as applied to depression in a sample of breast-cancer patients finishing cancer treatment and found that the "resilience" trajectory was most common (61% of participants). More recently, in a study of 125 cancer survivors, Bonanno's model was applied to newly diagnosed patients (Lotfi-Jam et al., 2019). Again, most survivors (80%) exhibited the "resilient" response, generally coping well over time, while 9% exhibited a "chronic" pattern of persistent distress over time. A "recovered" trajectory characterized 6% of the sample, with high initial distress that abated over time. Patients characterized by the remaining trajectory – "delayed," representing 5% of the survivors – coped well initially but struggled after completion of treatment. The good news about this study, and others like it, is that it shows us that most cancer survivors tolerate the course of cancer diagnosis and treatment without developing significant psychological difficulties. In individuals with cancer, resilience has been positively correlated with QoL and negatively correlated with depression (Maatouk et al., 2018; Popa-Velea et al., 2017).Nevertheless, a noteworthy minority of patients struggle after diagnosis, and for those individuals, psychological support can be helpful.

Common trajectories of distress for cancer patients include resilience, recovered, delayed, and chronic

1.4.3   Posttraumatic Growth

A concept related to resilience is posttraumatic growth (PTG), which was first defined by Tedeschi and Calhoun in 2004. PTG refers to growth after experiencing a traumatic event, which makes it different from resilience by suggesting that the individual improves as a result of their cancer experience (the "trauma" in this context), versus recovering baseline levels of functioning. While prevalence rates vary by type of cancer, in a sample of patients with different types of cancer, PTG was moderate to high in 20.5% (Liu et al., 2021). A recent systematic review found that most studies demonstrate a significant positive association between QoL and PTG in cancer survivors (Liu et al., 2020).

1.4.4   Survivorship

Survivorship can be complicated by late and persistent effects of treatment

As cancer survival rates increase (CDC, 2021), the length of cancer survivorship is also extended. Survivorship refers to an extended time that individuals diagnosed with cancer live with the physical and emotional sequelae of the disease and its treatment. There is a growing recognition of the persistent effects of cancer treatment as well as the late effects of cancer treatment. Examples of persistent effects include lymphedema, hormonal or fertility issues, fear of recurrence, fatigue, neuropathy, and cognitive difficulties ("chemobrain") (Cancer.Net, 2019). Examples of late effects include cataracts, heart or lung problems, and osteoporosis (National Cancer Institute (NCI), 2016).

The end of treatment can provoke anxiety in some individuals

While it is reasonable to think that the end of cancer treatment is a celebratory event (and indeed in some treatment settings, the last treatment is celebrated by the patient ringing a bell), sometimes this transition can provoke anxiety. Some survivors fear the loss of more frequent surveillance by and contact with their cancer team during treatment. The end of treatment leads some to consider the impact of cancer on their identities, relationships, and roles. Fear of cancer recurrence may increase as the perceived protective benefits of treatment fade.

1.5   Differential Diagnosis

The vegetative signs of depression in cancer settings include changes in appetite and/or weight, lack of energy, and changes in sleep. These same symptoms are commonly associated with cancer or cancer treatment. For example, taste changes associated with chemotherapy can lead to poor appetite and to weight loss. Hormonal changes associated with cancer in turn can be related to weight gain. Fatigue can be an early sign of cancer but is also a common side effect of both chemotherapy and radiation therapy. Steroid use in cancer treatment can interfere with sleep, as can worries about cancer or mortality. This overlap in symptoms can make the diagnosis of depression more complicated in the cancer setting. Some have advocated for a different methodology for diagnosing depression in the cancer setting, but no consensus has been established (Saracino et al., 2016).

1.6   Comorbidities

Sleep difficulties are common in the cancer setting. These may arise from the use of specific treatments (e.g., steroids) or from distressing symptoms (e.g., pain, nausea). Sleep difficulties are also a symptom of depression (either hypersomnia or insomnia) and a common symptom of anxiety. Many individuals with a cancer diagnosis talk about the nighttime being the worst time for them in terms of their worries, when there are fewer distractions. A cancer diagnosis can trigger worry (about mortality, upcoming scans, the effectiveness of treatment, existential issues), which can vary in intensity over the cancer trajectory.

Mild cognitive dysfunction has been documented in individuals treated for cancer (Palmer, 2020). Cognitive difficulties labeled "chemo-brain" or "chemo-fog" have also been associated with surgery, radiation therapy, and hormonal therapy.

1.7 Diagnostic Procedures and Documentation

1.7.1 Distress Screening

Distress screening has long been advocated in the cancer setting as a tool to identify those patients struggling to cope with their diagnosis or treatment (Adler et al., 2008). Because more than 1,500 cancer centers in the US are now accredited by the CoC, when distress screening became an accreditation standard, it became a common practice. The CoC standard allows for institutional latitude in terms of screening tool, frequency of screening, and setting for screening. The NCCN Distress Thermometer and Problem List (NCCN, 2021; see Appendix 3) is available for use without charge and is the most used screening tool, although it is not used universally. The Problem List includes sections on physical concerns, emotional concerns, practical concerns, social concerns, and spiritual concerns. Some research has suggested that the domain of emotional concerns is the second most common driver of distress in cancer patients, after physical symptoms (Deshields et al., 2018). As an aspirational goal, the NCCN advocates screening every patient at every visit to identify distress promptly. While many cancer centers struggle with more frequent screening, some consider this a hallmark of patient-centered care. The CoC and the NCCN advocate for a broad conceptualization of distress (see definition in Section 1.2.2; NCCN, 2021, p. DIS-1), which includes psychological manifestations as well as physical, social, and practical/financial problems. Distress screening can help to identify psychological difficulties in cancer patients as well as to identify patients who are struggling in other realms of functioning. An additional distress screening tool available to use without charge is the Patient Screening Questions for Supportive Care developed by the Coleman Foundation (Appendix 4).

> **Distress screening helps identify patients who are struggling with stressors that could be disruptive to their care**

1.7.2 Symptom Assessment

Symptom burden in cancer patients has been associated with poorer QoL and worse depression (Fitzgerald et al., 2015). In a study of 542 cancer patients, more than 90% of patients reported at least one symptom (Deshields et al., 2014), and QoL was negatively correlated with overall symptom burden. Prostate cancer patients had the lowest symptom burden, and colorectal cancer patients had the highest symptom burden.

Several common patient-reported symptom assessment tools include psychological symptoms. The most commonly used tools (all available for use without charge) are the Edmonton Symptom Assessment Scale (ESAS; Bruera et al., 1991), a 9-item tool that includes depression and anxiety; the Memorial

> **Symptom burden has been associated with poorer quality of life and worse depression**

Symptom Assessment Scale (MSAS; Portenoy et al., 1994), a 32-item measure that includes "feeling nervous," "feeling sad," "feeling irritable," and "worrying"; and the Patient Reported Outcomes Measurement Information System (PROMIS; Wagner et al., 2015), which has a question bank with questions assessing depression/sadness, anxiety/fear, anger, and positive affect/well-being.

1.7.3   Depression Assessment

Several measures are commonly used for assessing depression in the cancer setting. Arguably, the most frequently used one is the Patient Health Questionnaire (Kroenke et al., 2001), which is available for use without charge as a 9-item version (PHQ-9) or a 2-item version (PHQ-2). In the PHQ-9, the last question asks about suicidal thoughts, which can be useful clinically but which also requires a timely review and response. The Hospital Anxiety and Depression Scale (HADS; Snaith, 2003) is available for use with a fee, is designed for use in medical settings, and has two 7-item subscales focused on depression and anxiety. The PROMIS system has three short-form options for depression, all available for use without charge, with 4, 6, or 8 items. The PROMIS item bank has 30 items that can be used to construct questionnaires of various lengths for the assessment of depression. The computerized adaptive testing (CAT) version of PROMIS is available for use with charge but allows for the tailoring of questions based on individual responses. The PHQ-4 is a commonly used measure in the cancer setting (and available for use without charge), composed of four items, with the first two focused on depression and the last two focused on anxiety.

1.7.4   Anxiety Assessment

Several measures are commonly used for assessing anxiety in the cancer setting. The most common is the Generalized Anxiety Disorder – 7 Scale (GAD-7; Spitzer et al., 2006), which has 7 items and is available for use without charge. The HADS noted above also has a 7-item subscale for anxiety and is available for use with a fee. The PROMIS system has four short-form options for assessing anxiety, with 4, 6, 7, and 8 items, respectively, all available for use without charge. The PROMIS item bank has 22 items for the assessment of anxiety. As noted previously, the PHQ-4 is a commonly used measure in the cancer setting and available for use without charge. Of the four items, the last two are focused on anxiety.

1.7.5   Quality of Life (QoL)

QoL life assessment can document the impact of cancer on an individual as well as the impact of treatment

QoL assessment is commonly used in medical settings to document the impact of illness, but it is also increasingly being used to measure the impact of cancer treatment. The Functional Assessment of Chronic Illness Therapy (FACIT; Cella et al., 1993) and the European Organization for Research and Treatment of Cancer Quality of Life Questionnaire (EORTC-QLQ-C30; Fayers et al.,

2002) are cancer-specific tools, and both systems are available for use without charge. The FACIT-General has 27 items, grouped into four subscales: Physical Well-being, Social/Family Well-Being, Emotional Well-Being, and Functional Well-Being. The EORTC-QLQ-C30 has 30 items, with 5 functional scales (including emotional functioning), 3 symptom scales, and 6 single-item measures. The Short Form 36 (SF36; Ware & Sherbourne, 1992) is a general (i.e., not cancer specific) QoL measure that is also available for use without charge. It has 36 items and subscales for emotional well-being and physical well-being. There is an abbreviated version, the SF-12, which includes the same subscales.

2

Theories and Models

Psycho-oncology is a relatively young field. Dr. Jimmie Holland, the founding mother of psycho-oncology, established the first psychiatry clinical service in a cancer center, at Memorial Sloan-Kettering, in 1977. She was also involved in the founding of the International Psycho-Oncology Society in 1984 and the American Psychosocial Oncology Society in 1986. She published the first textbook *Psycho-Oncology* in 1989 and established the first journal devoted to the topic in 1992. Dr. Holland led the inaugural Distress Management Panel of the National Comprehensive Cancer Network in 1997; and this panel produced the first distress management guidelines in 1999. While relatively young, the field of psycho-oncology builds on traditions established in the fields of health psychology/behavioral medicine and consultation–liaison psychiatry.

2.1　Biopsychosocial Model of Cancer

Discourse on cancer care has long incorporated psychological factors. Beginning in the 1800s and extending into the early 20th century, the psychology of cancer largely centered on issues of fear, guilt, and shame, owing to a combination of stigmatization and fatalism (Fabrega, 1990). Cancer and the associated symptoms – both physical and emotional – were typically not discussed with patients to avoid contributing to a pervasive sense of hopelessness. Psychological dysfunction was viewed only as a consequence of cancer, rather than a factor impacting clinical course and care. For example, a survey of physicians published in 1961 indicated that only 10% would tell their patients about a terminal cancer diagnosis (Oken, 1961). Overwhelming fatalism about a cancer diagnosis relegated care of cancer patients to religious groups, and providers and family members were discouraged from disclosing a cancer diagnosis to affected patients to maintain hope and minimize emotional distress (Holland, 2010). The survey about communication preferences was repeated in 1977, and a major cultural shift was highlighted, with 97% of physicians at that time favoring telling a patient about their cancer diagnosis. The dramatic reversal was thought to be attributable to updates in medical school and hospital training, more clinical experience with cancer, improvements in cancer treatments, an increase in public awareness, and more personal experiences with cancer (Novack et al., 1979). The patient rights movement of the 1970s also helped to spur this change (Annas, 2017).

Prior to the 1970s, many physicians avoided informing patients of their cancer diagnoses.

In the mid-1900s, psychiatrists and many oncologists ascribed to psychodynamic formulations of cancer; traumatic life events and extreme personality factors were considered causal factors for the development of cancer. Ultimately, as both psychiatry and medicine advanced, psychosomatic medicine shifted away from its psychoanalytic orientation and toward two new fields that were particularly relevant to cancer care: psychoneuroimmunology (the study of the interaction between the mind, the nervous system, and immune function; Ader & Cohen, 1975), and consultation-liaison psychiatry (the diagnosis and management of psychiatric disorders that are comorbid with general/surgical illness). In both fields, researchers began using quantitative and translational research methods to measure biological events during cancer treatment and the associated stress, coping, and psychological burden. These studies aligned with Engel's biopsychosocial model (Engel, 1982), and the field moved away from a cause-effect model of disease and toward a model that includes psychosocial dimensions of a patient's experience (personal, emotional, family, community), in addition to biological aspects (disease). The biopsychosocial model has been applied to understanding issues of cancer prevention and development of cancer, management of cancer-related physical symptoms and adjustment to cancer, response to cancer treatment and survivorship, and end-of-life issues.

Psychoneuro-immunology and consultation-liaison psychiatry served as the foundation for psychosocial oncology

Researchers studying cancer prevention and early detection utilize the biopsychosocial framework to determine possible risk factors for developing cancer, and, in particular, to identify changeable risk factors. Cumulative evidence suggests that genetic, environmental, lifestyle, endocrine, and socioeconomic factors all play a role in the development of cancer (Colditz et al., 2006; Lutgendorf et al., 2010). Özkan et al. (2017) compared biological, psychological, and social risk factors between women with breast cancer and a control group. In addition to replicating previous studies examining reproductive factors and comorbidities, their data suggested that several factors were associated with an increased risk of breast cancer, including the existence of a major stressor in the last five years of the premorbid period, perception of inadequate social support, use of avoidance as a coping strategy, being a housewife, family history of cancer, advanced age, and higher BMI. Several studies examined the relationship between depression and cancer risk, with at least two meta-analyses suggesting a small and positive association between depression and the overall occurrence risk of cancer (Jia et al., 2017; Oerlemans et al., 2007) via a variety of indirect effects. For example, there is some evidence to suggest that recurrent emotional distress may diminish natural killer cell function, which is thought to play a role in tumor cell control (Kiecolt-Glaser et al., 2002). Similarly, symptoms of depression may contribute to hypothalamic-pituitary-adrenal (HPA) axis dysregulation, increase cortisol concentrations and associated inflammatory responses, as well as inhibit DNA repair, which collectively may inhibit defense processes for hormone-related cancers (Spiegel & Giese-Davis, 2003). Psychological distress is also associated with lifestyle-related risk factors for the development of cancer, such as smoking or overuse of other harmful substances, decreased physical activity, and less healthy diet. Psychosocial factors, including demographic and structural factors, cognitive variables, and

The biopsychosocial model has been applied to all aspects of cancer care, from cancer prevention to end-of-life

socioemotional variables, may also impact the likelihood of individuals participating in cancer screening (Magai et al., 2007), and therefore the stage at which cancer is detected.

Cancer-related pain is a particularly salient example of the biopsychosocial model

The biopsychosocial model is often used as a framework for examining cancer-related pain, and how pain impacts coping throughout the cancer journey (Novy & Aigner, 2014). A large body of literature demonstrates a correlation between higher levels of depression, anxiety, and distress, lower quality of life, and lack of social support with higher pain levels among cancer patients, even when controlling for disease type, disease stage, and treatment. Higher pain levels, in turn, can lead to changes in pain behaviors, such as inactivity, which can lead to deconditioning, greater likelihood of injury, and poorer immune function. These findings underscore the importance of multidisciplinary treatment throughout the treatment process.

Most frequently, the biopsychosocial framework is applied to issues related to coping with and response to treatment, survivorship, morbidity, and mortality. A robust literature identifies psychosocial and disease parameters that are predictors of or associated with disease progression, overall health status, and health-related quality of life (HRQOL) in cancer patients (Pikhart & Pikhartova, 2015). HRQOL has been identified as a potential predictor of survival in several disease groups, including colorectal (Braun et al., 2011), pancreatic (Braun et al., 2013), lung (Gupta et al., 2012), and breast cancers (Staren et al., 2011). Further, psychological distress has been linked to poorer outcomes in cancer patients via a variety of potential pathways, such as unhealthy lifestyle behaviors, poor treatment adherence, increased symptom burden and amplification of physical symptoms, additive functional impairment, increased utilization of medical resources, and higher morbidity and mortality. Recognition of psychosocial and environmental factors and their interplay with demographic factors and disease qualities has informed current standards of care (Institute of Medicine, 2013; NCCN, 2021) and helped to inform the creation of survivorship care plans that incorporate supportive interventions.

Psychological distress has been linked to poorer outcomes in cancer patients

Patients with greater psychological distress appear to have increased rates of death from selected cancers

The biopsychosocial framework has been applied to examining the predictive capacity of psychological distress concerning cancer mortality. The findings can be summarized as follows (Chida et al., 2008; Hamer et al., 2009):

- Individuals with more psychological distress appear to have increased rates of death from selected cancers relative to individuals with low distress, even when controlling for known risk factors for select malignancies, such as adverse health behaviors. This relationship appears to differ across disease sites.
- Stress-related psychosocial factors (e.g., more stressful life experiences, stress-prone personalities, unfavorable coping styles, emotional distress, poor QoL), adversely affect cancer survival and appear to be related to increased cancer mortality.
- The association between distress and incident cancer death is stronger for those with a previous cancer history. In patients without a cancer history, psychological distress appears to be associated with an increase in lung cancer mortality.

2.2   Models of Cancer-Related Distress

Distress in the cancer setting extends along a continuum, ranging from common, normal feelings of vulnerability, sadness, and fear to problems that can become disabling, such as depression, anxiety, panic, social isolation, and existential and spiritual crisis. In the Distress Management Guidelines, the NCCN (2021) also describes distress as arising from a combination of patient-level characteristics and periods of increased vulnerability (see Table 1).

The following sections offer an overview of models for the development of cancer-related distress.

Distress exists on a continuum from common feelings of sadness and fear to depression, anxiety, social isolation, and existential/ spiritual crisis

Table 1
Risk Factors for Distress and Periods of Increased Vulnerability Contribute to the Development of Cancer-Related Distress

Risk factors for distress	Periods of increased vulnerability
<ul><li>History of psychiatric disorder or SUD</li><li>History of depression/suicide attempt</li><li>Cognitive impairment</li><li>Communication barriers</li><li>Severe comorbid illness</li><li>Social issues:<ul><li>– Family/caregiver conflicts</li><li>– Inadequate social support</li><li>– Living alone</li><li>– Financial problems</li><li>– Limited access to medical care</li><li>– Young or dependent children</li><li>– Younger age</li><li>– History of abuse</li></ul></li><li>Spiritual/religious concerns</li><li>Uncontrolled symptoms</li><li>Cancer type associated with risk of depression</li><li>Diagnostic delay</li><li>Higher levels of preoperative anxiety and postoperative pain</li><li>Difficulty tolerating uncertainty</li></ul>	<ul><li>Finding a suspicious symptom</li><li>During diagnostic workup</li><li>Finding out the diagnosis</li><li>Learning about genetic/familial cancer risk</li><li>Awaiting treatment</li><li>Change in treatment modality</li><li>Significant treatment-related complications</li><li>End of treatment</li><li>Admission to/discharge from hospital</li><li>Transition to survivorship</li><li>Surveillance</li><li>Treatment failure</li><li>Recurrence/progression</li><li>Advanced cancer</li><li>End of life</li></ul>

Adapted from National Comprehensive Cancer Network (NCCN), 2021.

2.2.1   Cancer-Related Distress as an Adjustment Disorder

Li et al. (2010) offer a model of cancer-related distress as adjustment-related challenges which exist on a continuum from a normal stress response to an adjustment disorder. Consistent with the *Diagnostic and Statistical Manual of Mental Disorders* (American Psychiatric Association (APA), 2013) definition

Cancer-related distress has been conceptualized as an adjustment disorder

of an adjustment disorder, an aspect of the cancer (e.g., diagnosis, onset of symptoms, progression) precipitates symptoms of distress, which may persist until the stressor is attenuated or the person adapts. At times, the burden of the stressor may be greater than the individual's resources for coping, particularly in combination with the individual's baseline vulnerabilities. Biological and psychosocial stressors interact to contribute to the development of distress, and this relationship is thought to be moderated by individual or interpersonal factors.

2.2.2   Self-Regulatory Model of Illness Behavior

When confronted with cancer, individuals attempt to assign meaning to the cancer through their perceptions about it – these perceptions influence psychological well-being

Several studies examined one or more components of the self-regulatory model of illness behavior (SRM; Leventhal et al., 1980) to predict distress in cancer populations. SRM has been applied to understanding how distress arises in some individuals with cancer but not in others. SRM provides a framework for examining the cognitive, behavioral, and perceptual processes that contribute to an individuals' initiation and maintenance of behaviors for managing health issues and associated adjustment outcomes (Leventhal et al., 2016). The SRM suggests that, when someone is confronted with an illness such as cancer, they attempt to assign meaning to the cancer through their perceptions about the illness, and those perceptions in turn influence psychological well-being (Dempster & McCorry, 2012). Relevant perceptions fall into several possible domains: timeline of the illness (how long it will last), perceived seriousness or consequences, the ability to cure or control the disease, the extent to which the disease makes sense to the person, the perceived cause, and the extent to which a person identifies as having the disease. Perceptions further influence coping responses, and patients may utilize strategies that fall into broad categorical styles of coping: emotion-oriented coping (regulating the emotional response to the stressors), and problem-oriented coping (managing the stressor or solving a cancer-related problem). Illness perceptions interact with coping styles to impact psychological well-being (Dempster et al., 2015). For example, when patients perceive their disease to be controllable and to have less serious consequences, they tend to use adaptive cognitive coping strategies such as problem-solving and re-appraisal. Similarly, when patients have high perceived control and utilize a problem-oriented coping style, they tend to have the lowest levels of anxiety/depression.

When patients have less dire perceptions of their disease, they tend to apply more adaptive coping strategies

Coping style appears to mediate the relationship between illness perceptions and cancer-related distress

Gibbons et al. (2016) examined the mediating effects of coping style on the relationship between illness perception and greater cancer-related distress in women with newly diagnosed breast cancer. Several illness perceptions were related to cancer-related distress, including the belief that the cancer or treatment effects would last longer, the belief about more severe consequences of the cancer, more identification with the illness, and less illness coherence. However, these effects were significant only when women also utilized anxious preoccupation as a passive coping strategy, thus lending support to a model in which coping style mediates the relationship between illness perceptions and cancer-related distress.

2.2.3   Stressful Life Events and the Impact of Coping Style on Cancer-Related Distress

Holland (2010) revised the original model of stress and coping (Park & Folkman, 1997) to conceptualize coping with cancer. When faced with a stressful life event (SLE) such as cancer, individuals appraise the situation based on pre-existing beliefs and goals. If global meaning and situational meaning are incongruent, the individual experiences heightened distress and attempts to apply a coping strategy. Whether or not the coping style is adaptive predicts subsequent adjustment or further distress. Adjustment requires acceptance or reappraisal (adjusting situational and/or global meaning) of the stressor.

Langford et al. (2017) evaluated whether coping style (e.g., adaptive versus maladaptive) mediates the relationship between SLEs and cancer-related distress. The data suggested that lower functional status and higher level of comorbidity predicted a greater number of SLEs and a greater impact of SLEs on current distress. As hypothesized, utilizing a maladaptive coping style (e.g., avoidance, denial, self-blame) was strongly associated with cancer-related distress. Further, maladaptive coping completely mediated the relationship between SLEs and distress. In other words, the use of maladaptive coping was thought to explain the relationship between SLEs and cancer-related distress, suggesting that coping style may be a particularly important target for intervention.

A robust body of literature examines the relationship between coping styles and the development of cancer-related distress, with maladaptive coping consistently predicting higher levels of distress and worse QoL. Meanwhile, adaptive coping (e.g., active coping, positive reframing, utilization of emotional support, acceptance, humor) has been linked to less distress and better adjustment to cancer (Shapiro et al., 2010). Similarly, exposure to SLEs has been linked not only to greater cancer-related distress, but also to better adjustment, which appears to be related to a greater likelihood of utilizing adaptive coping strategies or to the patient's ability to identify positive outcomes resulting from the stressful event (Shand et al., 2015).

Brennan (2001) proposed a social-cognitive transition (SCT) model of adjustment to cancer that incorporates several of the aforementioned constructs: cancer as a major stressor, coping with and adjustment to cancer as processes, and posttraumatic stress versus posttraumatic growth (PTG). Like Park and Folkman (1997), who saw coping as a process, Brennan highlighted the utility of examining adjustment to cancer as a process rather than a state to be achieved. The SCT model provides a framework within which individual differences in cancer adjustment can be understood. The model proposes that individuals have an "assumptive world," which is a representation of the world that reflects cultural and social contexts and the accumulation of our life experiences. When we have expectations about ourselves or the world based on our assumptions, those assumptions are either confirmed or disconfirmed based on a subsequent experience, such as a cancer diagnosis. If the expectation is confirmed, the assumption is strengthened; if the expectation is disconfirmed, there is likely to be a period of stress, during which we incorporate new data that inform the adjustment of the baseline assumption. The time needed to adjust assumptions is seen as the adjustment period and may be characterized by the use of adaptive or maladaptive coping strategies.

Models are a useful tool for understanding the complex factors that contribute to a patient's experience with cancer. We expect that models of health status across the cancer continuum, models of psychological distress, and models of care will continue to evolve as the field develops.

3

Diagnosis and Treatment Indications

3.1　Distress in Cancer

Distress is associated with reduced adherence to treatment, increased frequency of medical encounters (acute care, emergency room, office visits), increased length of hospital stays, poorer QoL, and reduced survival (NCCN, 2021). The etiology of distress in cancer is multifactorial and related to the significant life changes associated with a serious illness. Many patients experience changes to employment causing financial, familial, and housing distress. Other patients experience significant physical complications of their disease as well as side effects and long-term sequelae of cancer treatment. These symptoms can occur at any time during the cancer continuum, including upon diagnosis, during the planning and initiation of cancer treatment, during adjustments to the treatment plan, and during remission and survivorship.

The CoC accreditation standard is very general and leaves much room for institutional decision-making about screening. The American Psychosocial Oncology Society (APOS), the Association of Oncology Social Workers (AOSW), and the Oncology Nursing Society (ONS) published a joint consensus on guidelines for distress screening and distress management (Pirl et al., 2014). The consensus statement included these recommendations:

1. A universal definition of distress among CoC-accredited programs. The organizations favored the NCCN definition of distress.
2. Validated instruments for distress screening, using published threshold values and ranges.
3. Screening instruments that are broadly focused rather than unidimensional.
4. Repeated screening versus one-time only.
5. Timely review of screening results.
6. For positive screens, identification of the cause of distress and triage to an appropriate clinician.

Several tools can be utilized for distress screening. The NCCN Distress Thermometer (DT) and Problem List (PL) (NCCN, 2021) is the most widely used brief general screening tool. The most common cutoff score for a positive screen is a score of 4 or more on the DT; the PL can provide additional information about contributors to a patient's distress, but a more detailed assessment may be needed to triage a patient to relevant resources. One example of a comprehensive distress screener is the Coleman Foundation Supportive Care Screening Tool. Other potential screening tools are mentioned below. Once distress has been identified, a variety of psychosocial interventions has proved efficacious in relieving distress and improving QoL.

Psychosocial interventions were also found to improve patient outcomes. The timing of specific interventions at specific points in the diagnosis-treatment-remission continuum may lead to greater efficacy. Psychoeducation is often most effective during the medical work-up and diagnosis phase. For patients in later stages of treatment with emerging distress, group therapy can be beneficial by giving patients a context for their experiences and the opportunity to process them with peers. Cognitive-behavioral techniques may be most beneficial during periods of extended treatment, though they can be used with patients at any stage in the cancer continuum. Examples of relevant specific cognitive-behavioral techniques are described later in this book (Chapter 4). Patients have increased vulnerability to distress during pivotal points in the cancer continuum (NCCN, 2021), including the investigation and diagnosis of their disease, receiving news about metastatic disease, awaiting treatment, the onset or increase of symptom burden, treatment-related complications, changes in the level of care (inpatient admission or discharge), treatment failure, completion of treatment, follow-up surveillance, survivorship transitions, recurrence of disease, and end-of-life care. The primary aim of psychosocial intervention is to reduce distress and improve outcomes.

3.2   Adjustment Disorders

Adjustment disorders are distinguished from distress by the presence of impaired functioning

According to the DSM-5 (APA, 2013), adjustment disorder occurs in response to an identifiable stressor. To justify the diagnosis of adjustment disorder, the patient must be experiencing significant psychological or behavioral distress beyond what otherwise might be expected in response to the identifiable stressor. The symptoms must occur within 3 months of the onset of the stressor and must lead to impairment in psychosocial domains (e.g., work, school, relationships). The symptoms should not persist beyond 6 months after the stressor is terminated. If the symptoms persist, other diagnoses must be considered. Patients may present with depressed mood, anxiety, or disturbance of conduct.

Adjustment disorders can present with depression, anxiety, disturbance of conduct, or any combination of these symptoms

Adjustment disorders may also be present with a combination of symptoms including mixed anxiety and depressed mood and mixed emotions and disturbance of conduct. Adjustment disorder is a psychological diagnosis that is differentiated from distress by the severity of symptoms and the presence of significant functional impairment. Patients may react in a wide variety of ways to the diagnosis and treatment of cancer, and often these reactions are expected and appropriate to the circumstances. However, in adjustment disorder, the patient's reactions and emotions interfere with their daily functioning, which may result in difficulties participating in cancer treatment. Clinicians should be aware that patients experiencing an adjustment disorder are at greater risk for suicide than the general population.

Adjustment disorders may be viewed as milder forms of other psychiatric disorders, even though the presenting symptoms do not otherwise meet the criteria for another disorder. The differential diagnosis for adjustment disorder with depressed mood, for example, includes major depressive disorder; the differential diagnosis for adjustment disorder with anxiety includes GAD and panic disorder. In addition to the differential diagnoses already listed, the differential diagnosis of adjustment disorders with mixed features (mixed anxiety and depressed mood or mixed disturbance of emotions and conduct) includes acute stress disorder and posttraumatic stress disorder (PTSD). It is important to establish the diagnosis of adjustment disorder versus an alternative mental-health disorder because responsiveness to treatment varies depending on the diagnosis. For example, patients with major depression or GAD are more likely to benefit from medication management or psychotherapy, whereas the evidence for these treatments in adjustment disorders is less robust. A thorough diagnostic interview is the most useful way to distinguish between the diagnoses. The interview may be complemented by clinical rating scales to screen for the presence of other mental-health disorders.

It is important to remember that the presence of cancer and the side effects of treatment may mimic mental-health symptoms. As noted previously, it is common for patients to experience fatigue, changes in energy level, changes in appetite, changes in sleep patterns, and changes in concentration because of their malignancy or associated treatments. The astute clinician recognizes these symptoms and further explores their underlying etiology to differentiate between cancer-associated symptoms, adjustment disorder, or other mood and anxiety disorders. If we take the example of appetite changes, a patient may experience loss of appetite secondary to changes in taste; difficulty swallowing; the presence of nausea, vomiting, diarrhea, or constipation; or alterations in anatomy secondary to surgical interventions. They may also have a loss of appetite as part of a syndrome of depression, where the actual desire to eat is profoundly diminished. At times, it is impossible to differentiate between symptoms of the underlying disease and symptoms of a psychological diagnosis. In these instances, the clinician should err on the side of caution and treat these symptoms as part of the diagnostic criteria of a mental-health disorder to avoid missing an opportunity to provide relief to a suffering patient.

> Some symptoms of cancer and associated treatments can overlap with the diagnostic criteria for mental illness

An adjustment disorder may be present in up to 19% of cancer patients (van Beek et al., 2019). The onset of adjustment disorder can occur at any time during the cancer continuum but is most likely during transition points, where new stressors ensue. A patient may also suffer from serial adjustment disorders when the symptoms abate with treatment but return in the presence of a new stressor.

Potential interventions for adjustment disorder include behavioral activation, supportive psychotherapy, cognitive-behavioral therapy (CBT), and associated therapies (described in Section 4.1). In general, in the absence of other comorbid mental-health diagnoses, the use of medication is limited in this population. For example, antidepressants have not consistently been shown to improve symptoms of adjustment disorder. For patients with adjustment disorder with anxiety-related distress who do not meet the criteria for an anxiety disorder, antihistaminergic medications (e.g., hydroxyzine), low-dose benzodiazepines, and hypnotics or sleep aids may provide temporary relief. The use of these medications should be time-limited and should support psychotherapeutic treatment modalities. Patients should be coached about the short-term benefits of medication and informed that psychological interventions have the greatest efficacy. The primary aim of treatment is to alleviate the symptoms specific to the adjustment disorder.

> Psychological interventions are the treatment of choice for adjustment disorder

> There is limited benefit for the use of medication in the treatment of adjustment disorders

3.3   Major Depressive Disorder

According to the DSM-5 (APA, 2013), major depressive disorder is diagnosed when patients experience a cluster of symptoms which include alterations in sleep, mood, energy, motivation, and concentration. Patients may experience reduced self-worth, feelings of guilt or low self-esteem, and may demonstrate poor self-care. Other symptoms associated with depression can include irritability, anger, crying spells, helplessness, hopelessness, increased aggression, increased reports of pain or other somatic symptoms, and sexual dysfunction. When depression is severe, patients may experience psychotic symptoms, such as hallucinations or delusions. Patients may also experience suicidal ideation and are at greater risk for self-harm and suicide attempts. (For further reading on the specific diagnostic criteria, readers are encouraged to reference the DSM-5 directly.) The underlying etiology of major depressive disorder is a combination of environmental and biological factors. Examples of environmental factors include socioeconomic status, employment, and level of social support; examples of biological factors include age, genetic predisposition and family history, cognitive functioning, presence of medical or psychiatric diagnoses, uncontrolled symptoms (pain, fatigue, anorexia, nausea, etc.), medications and supplements, physical activity, sleep, diet, and drug and alcohol use. For patients with cancer, the presence of the malignancy may create both biological and environmental factors that lead to the onset of major depression. The prevalence of major depression in patients with cancer is estimated to be up to 24% (Krebber et al., 2014).

> Cancer causes many biological risk factors for the development of a major depressive episode

> Major depression can be triggered by stressful events during the patient's experience with cancer

The differential diagnosis for major depressive disorder is broad, but for patients with cancer most commonly includes depression secondary to a general medical condition, adjustment disorder with depressed mood, PTSD, substance-induced mood disorder, apathy, and demoralization. Major depression is differentiated from distress in cancer when patients with cancer meet the DSM diagnostic criteria, which are more specific. It is differentiated from adjustment disorder when the symptoms affecting the patient are present with the frequency and timing described above, and when symptoms are not necessarily, but may be, temporally associated with a specific event (e.g., cancer diagnosis). As with adjustment disorder, there can be some symptomatic overlap between symptoms of major depression and symptoms related to malignancy and the side effects of treatment for malignancy. The most common overlapping symptoms include changes in energy, appetite, sleep, cognitive functioning, or concentration. Major depression can be further described based on severity. The categories of mild, moderate, or severe are based on the number of symptoms present, the severity of the symptoms, and the degree to which these symptoms cause disability.

The most commonly used screening tool for depression is the PHQ-9, with recommended cutoffs of 5 for mild, 10 for moderate, 15 for moderately severe, and 20 for severe depression (Kroenke et al., 2001). Other useful screening tools include the Beck Depression Inventory-II (Beck et al., 1996) and the Hospital Anxiety and Depression Scale (14 items total, 7-item subscale for depression; Zigmond & Snaith, 1983). The score on these rating scales helps to further define the severity of the depressive episode.

Risk factors for a depressive episode are similar to the risk factors previously identified for distress in cancer. The greatest risk factor for the onset of a depressive episode is a history of previous depressive episodes. Cancer-related risk factors include poor prognosis/advanced disease and symptom burden (particularly pain, fatigue, and nausea).

The primary aim of treatment is the remission of the depressive episode. Remission can be measured objectively with serial depression questionnaires and repeating the diagnostic interview with the patient. The treatment plan should be guided by the severity of the major depression. For example, patients with mild to moderate symptoms may experience equal or greater symptom relief with psychotherapy compared to psychotherapy plus medication or medication alone. For patients with moderate to severe depression, medication should strongly be considered as part of the treatment plan. Aggressive treatment is recommended for patients with severe or life-threatening major depression (accompanied by suicidal ideation or catatonia), and medication, psychotherapy, and psychiatric hospitalization may all be indicated. Untreated and undertreated depression leads to worse QoL for the patient, worse medical outcomes, increased healthcare utilization and cost, and increased provider distress (McFarland et al., 2019; Satin et al., 2009). Large placebo-controlled trials involving patients with cancer are generally lacking, and those that exist have been reviewed as generally having low-quality evidence (Ostuzzi et al., 2018). The data concerning which medication to choose is based primarily on clinical trials in the general population and the physician's clinical judgment. More details on medications can be found in Table 2 in Chapter 4.

Multiple factors and conditions contribute to the ability of treatment providers to help patients reach treatment goals. The presence of comorbid psychological and psychiatric conditions may contribute to reduced treatment responsiveness. The severity and type of cancer also increase the risk of developing major depression and increase the difficulty of treating a major depressive episode. Cancer and the associated treatments cause a hyperinflammatory state that contributes to depressive symptoms and may also make depressive symptoms more difficult to treat. Upon remission of major depression, symptoms can recur at any point along the cancer continuum. As stated above, total remission is the goal of a treatment since partial remission leaves the patient at greater risk for recurrence of a depressive episode. Patients benefit from ongoing screening for recurrent symptoms and aggressive management of these symptoms to mitigate poor outcomes.

The treatment goal for any mental illness is the full remission of symptoms, though this can be difficult to achieve

Patients with moderate to severe depression likely need a combination of psychotherapy and medication management

Cancer is an inflammatory disease that can predispose patients to depression or make depression harder to treat

3.4 Anxiety Disorders

3.4.1 Generalized Anxiety Disorder (GAD)

According to the DSM-5 (APA, 2013), GAD is diagnosed as the presence of excessive anxiety and worry occurring most days for at least 6 months. Such excessive anxiety or worry should involve multiple life domains such as health, family, employment, education, and finances. This worry is difficult to control and can be associated with problems with energy, focus, concentra-

All stages of cancer can induce severe anxiety

tion, and sleep. Patients often experience increased irritability and an inability to settle down or feel calm. (For further reading on the specific diagnostic criteria, readers are encouraged to reference the DSM-5 directly.) The differential diagnosis for GAD is broad, but for patients with cancer, it commonly includes anxiety because of a general medical condition, adjustment disorder with anxious features, panic disorder, and anxiety related to medication effects or substance abuse. The prevalence of GAD in patients with cancer can run as high as 17% (Mitchell et al., 2011). All stages of the cancer continuum can induce high levels of anxiety and are risk factors for the onset or exacerbation of GAD. The most common screening tool for GAD is the GAD-7 (Spitzer et al., 2006), which has seven items, with cutoffs of 5 for mild anxiety, 10 for moderate anxiety, and 15 for severe anxiety. Other commonly used tools include the PROMIS anxiety scale (Wagner et al., 2015) and the HADS (14 items total, 7-item subscale for anxiety; Snaith, 2003).

GAD is differentiated from adjustment disorder with anxiety based on the patient presenting with complaints of anxiety and meeting the diagnostic criteria outlined in the DSM-5. In general, GAD is more severe and debilitating than adjustment disorder with anxiety. Treatment of GAD should be directed by symptom severity and based on the willingness of the patient to engage in the specific treatment modality. Psychotherapy is the treatment of choice for most cases of GAD. For mild to moderate cases, psychotherapy alone may be sufficient to achieve remission. However, in moderate to severe cases, patients likely need psychotherapy with medication to achieve remission of symptoms, which is the primary goal of treatment. As is the case with the previously discussed mental-health conditions, treatment for the remission of symptoms is made more difficult by psychiatric comorbidity and the presence of psychosocial stressors. Even when symptoms have remitted, they may recur at any stage of the cancer continuum. Therefore, ongoing surveillance and aggressive treatment of recurrent symptoms are priorities.

Patients with moderate to severe generalized anxiety disorder should be offered psychotherapy and medication

A subset of the patients who experience GAD has concurrent episodes of panic attacks. The presence of panic attacks necessarily changes the approach to the management of GAD, requiring specific strategies to mitigate panic attacks in addition to GAD. Panic attacks are described in the next section.

Patients with generalized anxiety disorder may also have panic attacks or agoraphobia

Another subset of patients who experience GAD has concurrent agoraphobia. According to the DSM-5 (APA, 2013), individuals with agoraphobia are fearful and anxious about two or more of the following situations: using public transportation, being in open spaces, being in enclosed places, standing in line or being in a crowd, or being outside of the home alone. The individual fears these situations because of overwhelming thoughts that escape might be difficult or help might not be available if they develop panic-like symptoms or other incapacitating or embarrassing symptoms. These situations almost always induce fear or anxiety and are often avoided or require the presence of a companion. Agoraphobia in patients with cancer may also be described as fear of being in a situation in which they could not easily receive medical attention if they had a medical emergency. It can also be a deterrent to getting treatment because of anxiety in the clinical setting. Agoraphobia can be a separate psychiatric diagnosis or can be a feature of GAD. The recommended treatment for agoraphobia with or without GAD is psychotherapy. Multiple psychotherapeutic modalities have been validated for the treatment of agoraphobia, including relaxation strategies, mindfulness-based techniques, cognitive-behavioral treatment, and acceptance and commitment therapy.

3.4.2   Panic Disorder

According to the DSM-5 (APA, 2013), panic disorder is diagnosed when there are recurrent and sudden panic attacks. These attacks are accompanied by an overwhelming sense of fear or dread. Sometimes patients describe a fear that they are about to die. The symptoms often escalate quickly and are usually self-limited. Physical symptoms of panic attacks include dizziness, lightheadedness, shortness of breath, choking sensation, heart racing or pain in the chest, diaphoresis, tremor or shakiness, gastrointestinal distress, and emotional or physical numbing or detachment. Over time, patients can develop a fear of future panic attacks that can, in turn, trigger more panic attacks. Patients will also go to great lengths to avoid potential triggers of panic attacks. (For further reading on the specific diagnostic criteria, readers are encouraged to reference the DSM-5 directly.) The differential diagnosis for panic disorder includes adjustment disorder with anxiety, GAD, PTSD, substance-induced anxiety disorder, and agoraphobia.

Panic attacks can occur in multiple psychiatric conditions and are not exclusive to panic disorder

Patients with cancer may experience high levels of anxiety and panic attacks at the time of diagnosis, during treatment, during ongoing survivorship care, or during recurrence. Panic attacks are initially most likely triggered by external events such as awaiting results of surveillance imaging or blood tests, or while undergoing chemotherapy or radiation; when severe, they may be triggered by any contact with a medical professional. Panic attacks become panic disorders when they begin to occur suddenly and without the presence of a trigger or warning, or when the fear of panic attacks begins to lead to panic attacks. This may lead to avoiding the medical setting altogether, which in turn can delay diagnosis, treatment, and surveillance and put the patient at risk of negative outcomes.

The prevalence of panic disorder in patients with cancer is estimated to be 9–20% (Osório et al., 2015; Slaughter et al., 2000), and the diagnosis is made based on clinical interview. The Patient Health Questionnaire – Panic Disorder Module (Kroenke et al., 2001) has been validated as a screening tool for panic disorder in this population. Panic disorder is differentiated from panic attacks associated with other psychiatric diagnoses when the patient has persistent worry specifically about panic attacks or their consequences, and/or the patient significantly changes their behavior to avoid situations that may induce a panic attack. Panic disorder may be comorbid with other psychiatric diagnoses.

Treatment of panic disorder should be guided by the frequency of panic attacks and severity of the disorder as well as by the willingness of the patient to engage in specific treatment modalities. Psychotherapy is an effective treatment for panic disorder. For individuals with frequent and severe panic episodes, medication can often support treatment and enable the patient to engage in psychotherapy. Selective serotonin reuptake inhibitors (SSRIs) and benzodiazepines are the medications of choice for panic disorder. Off-label use of hydroxyzine as needed can take the place of benzodiazepines for patients

Medications can be offered for panic disorder to supplement or enable participation in psychotherapy

with a contraindication to benzodiazepine treatment. The primary goal of treatment is remission of symptoms, but this is made more difficult when there is psychiatric comorbidity or the presence of psychosocial stressors. Even when symptoms have remitted, they may recur at any stage of the cancer continuum; therefore, ongoing surveillance and aggressive treatment of recurrent symptoms is especially important.

3.4.3   Specific Phobias

Per the DSM-5 (APA, 2013), phobias are diagnosed when there is "marked fear or anxiety about a specific object or situation." In addition, the fear is persistent, and the affected individual works very hard to avoid the feared stimulus. Phobias can be successfully treated with cognitive-behavioral approaches, but in an acute situation, anxiolytic medication may be needed.

Some phobias can be particularly problematic in the cancer setting. Perhaps the most obvious is a needle phobia, which can complicate treatment by making blood draws difficult, or by increasing distress around chemotherapy administration. Claustrophobia can be an issue when an MRI is a needed tool for disease surveillance. It can also be an issue for administration of radiation therapy for head/neck cancers, when the head is immobilized with a mask secured to the table (Nixon et al., 2019). Germ phobia can be problematic for some patients who are immunocompromised due to their cancer treatment.

3.5   Trauma-Related Disorders

3.5.1   Acute Stress Disorder

Acute stress disorder starts within 3 days of a stressors and is limited to 1 month following a stressor

According to the DSM-5 (APA, 2013), acute stress disorder occurs in response to directly experiencing severe physical trauma or sexual violence, witnessing traumatic events, learning of a traumatic event from a close contact, or frequently being exposed to intense details of a traumatic event. Acute stress disorder is a complex diagnosis requiring the presence of 9 or more symptoms across five symptom categories as outlined in the DSM-5. In general, acute stress disorder is a cluster of symptoms which include mood disturbance, recurring memories or dreams of the event, distress when presented with reminders of the event and efforts to avoid reminders, and feelings of physical or emotional detachment. Patients may also experience problems with sleep, focus, irritability, and anger, as well as fear that another traumatic event may occur. (For further reading on the specific diagnostic criteria, readers are encouraged to reference the DSM-5 directly.) The symptoms of acute stress disorder last between 3 days and 1 month and are expected to resolve. If symptoms persist beyond 1 month, an alternate diagnosis must be explored.

The differential diagnosis for acute stress disorder is broad, but in this patient population, it most commonly includes adjustment disorder, PTSD, panic disorder, GAD, and major depressive disorder. Acute stress disorder may also present as a comorbid condition with any other psychiatric diagnosis. The prevalence of acute stress disorder in patients with cancer may be as high as 33% (Pedersen & Zachariae, 2010). The diagnosis of acute stress disorder is made based upon clinical interviews. A potential screening tool for acute stress disorder is the Stanford Acute Stress Reaction Questionnaire.

Acute stress disorder is differentiated from alternative diagnoses based on the patient meeting criteria for a cluster of symptoms in each of the symptom categories. Acute stress disorder is differentiated from PTSD by the duration of symptoms, which are limited to 1 month. The onset of acute stress disorder often precedes PTSD, though there is no direct progression from one diagnosis to the next. Up to 53% of patients with cancer who develop acute stress disorder develop PTSD (Pedersen & Zachariae, 2010). Up to 36% of patients ultimately diagnosed with PTSD do not meet the criteria for acute stress disorder within the first month of their cancer diagnosis (Pedersen & Zachariae). Risk factors for developing acute stress disorder in the cancer setting include female sex, younger age at cancer diagnosis, lack of social support, and poor communication with the treatment team. Although these symptoms may occur at any time along the cancer continuum, patients are particularly vulnerable during transitional events such as: upon learning of their diagnosis, of disease relapse, of disease progression; when treatment options have been exhausted; immediately prior to or following surgery; during or after receiving treatment for their disease, or any hospitalization for complications of their disease or treatment; and at the end of life.

The treatment of acute stress disorder includes multiple psychotherapeutic modalities. Medication has limited utility in the treatment of acute stress disorder, except in the presence of a comorbid diagnosis (depression, anxiety, panic disorder, etc.). The primary goal of treatment is the full remission of symptoms. As is the case with the previously discussed mental-health conditions, achieving remission of symptoms is rendered more difficult by psychiatric comorbidity and the presence of psychosocial stressors. Even when symptoms have remitted, they may recur at any stage of the cancer continuum; therefore, ongoing surveillance and aggressive treatment of recurrent symptoms is paramount.

Psychotherapy is the treatment of choice for acute stress disorder

3.5.2   Posttraumatic Stress Disorder

According to the DSM-5 (APA, 2013), PTSD occurs in response to directly experiencing severe physical trauma or sexual violence, witnessing traumatic events, learning of a traumatic event from a close contact, or frequently experiencing extreme exposure to details of a traumatic event. Similar to acute stress disorder, PTSD is a complex psychiatric diagnosis requiring multiple symptoms in multiple domains. In general PTSD is a cluster of symptoms which includes experiencing negative emotions and worldview, cognitive distortions regarding the traumatic event, significant effort to avoid reminders of the trauma, and frequent memories and dreams of the trauma which trigger negative emotional states. Patients may experience problems with sleep, focus, memory, irritability and anger, and may act in dangerous ways. The symptoms must have lasted for longer than 1 month and must cause significant distress or impairment. (For further reading on the specific diagnostic criteria, readers are encouraged to reference the DSM-5 directly.)

Posttraumatic stress disorder is diagnosed after symptoms have been present for 1 month

The differential diagnosis for PTSD is broad, but in this patient population most commonly includes adjustment disorder, acute stress disorder, panic disorder, GAD, and major depressive disorder. PTSD may also present as a comorbid condition with any other psychiatric diagnosis. The prevalence of PTSD in patients with cancer may be as high as 14% (Cordova et al., 2017). The diagnosis of PTSD is made based on the clinical interview. Multiple screening tools exist to identify patients at risk for PTSD. The PC-PTSD is a 5-item, self-administered screening tool that can be used in this patient population. If a patient screens positive (responding "yes" to 3 of the 5 items), further assessment with a diagnostic interview is warranted to confirm or exclude the diagnosis. PTSD is differentiated from alternative diagnoses based on the patient meeting criteria for a cluster of symptoms across each of the symptom categories. PTSD is differentiated from acute stress disorder based on the specific symptom criteria being met and the presence of symptoms for greater than 1 month from the stressful event. Risk factors for the development of PTSD in the cancer setting include a history of trauma before the cancer diagnosis, a history of PTSD before the cancer diagnosis, lower socioeconomic status, younger age, limited social support, and advanced or aggressive cancer diagnosis.

Similar to acute stress disorder, the symptoms of PTSD may occur at any time along the cancer continuum. Like acute stress disorder, patients are particularly vulnerable during transitional events including upon learning their diagnosis, immediately prior to or following surgery, after repetitive exposure to cancer treatments (e.g., chemotherapy, radiation therapy, transfusions, photopheresis), during or after any hospitalization for complications of their disease or treatment, upon learning of relapsed disease, upon learning that their disease has advanced and all treatment options have been exhausted, and at the end of life.

CBT and its trauma-specific variants have the greatest evidence base for treatment of PTSD

The treatment of PTSD includes multiple psychotherapeutic modalities, particularly CBT and its trauma-specific variants, such as prolonged exposure and cognitive processing therapy. Other treatments include eye movement desensitization and reprocessing (EMDR) and stress inoculation training. Medication is useful for treating severe mood or anxiety symptoms or for the treatment of comorbid diagnoses. As always, the primary goal of treatment is the full remission of symptoms. As with the previously discussed mental-health conditions, treatment to remission of symptoms is made more difficult by the presence of psychiatric comorbidity and psychosocial stressors. Even when symptoms have remitted, they may recur at any stage of the cancer continuum; therefore, ongoing surveillance and aggressive treatment of recurrent symptoms is important.

3.6   Cognitive Dysfunction Secondary to Cancer Treatment

Cognitive dysfunction secondary to cancer treatment presents with a wide array and combination of deficits in various cognitive domains (Asher & Myers, 2015). This syndrome, often termed "chemo-brain" or "chemo-fog," is an increasingly recognized phenomenon occurring along the cancer continuum. Common symptoms of cognitive dysfunction are:

- Increasing forgetfulness
- Reduced processing speed
- Impaired concentration
- Reduced ability to sustain attention
- Reduced ability to multitask
- Problems with word-finding
- Reduced reaction time
- Short-term memory impairment

Patients rarely experience long-term memory deficits, new deficits in reasoning or problem solving, aphasia, agnosia, or apraxia. Cognitive dysfunction secondary to cancer treatment is a complicated diagnosis as symptoms may overlap with other clinical syndromes. The differential diagnosis includes fatigue and deconditioning, disordered sleep, uncontrolled pain, depression, anxiety disorders, side effects of nonchemotherapy medication (opiates, corticosteroids, benzodiazepines, etc.), other underlying medical problems (thyroid abnormalities, anemia, liver dysfunction, renal dysfunction), and nutritional deficits. Further complicating this diagnosis is the fact that some patients may have had pre-existing cognitive impairment that was previously unidentified. These patients may have a comorbid diagnosis of cognitive impairment that is inappropriately attributed to cancer treatments. Some patients may also have subsyndromal or mild cognitive impairment before treatment that was exacerbated by cancer treatments. For example, 20–35% of patients with breast cancer were found to have pre-existing cognitive impairment compared to their peers (Asher & Myers, 2015). Therefore, cognitive dysfunction secondary to cancer treatments remains a diagnosis of exclusion after other potentially reversible diagnoses have been investigated and ruled out. It is important to remember that there may also be two or more processes active at the same time.

If possible, screen for cognitive dysfunction prior to treatment to determine a baseline for posttreatment evaluation

Up to 75% of patients may experience a degree of cognitive impairment during their cancer treatment (Asher & Myers, 2015). As many as 35% of those patients may have persistent deficits lasting months to years, which suggests that the cognitive deficits may be reversible over time but a substantial number of patients may live with long-term or permanent deficits. Therefore, it is important to screen patients for the emergence of cognitive impairment.

Most patients with cancer experience at least mild symptoms of cognitive impairment

Although no gold-standard screening tool exists for screening patients with cancer for cognitive impairment, several validated tools for screening in the general patient population are available, including the Mini-Mental Status Exam (MMSE), the Montreal Cognitive Assessment (MOCA), the St. Louis University Mental Status Exam (SLUMS), and the Mini-Cog. Three options for self-reported cognitive impairment exist for patients with cancer: the Attentional Function Index, the Patient Reported Outcomes Measurement and Information System (PROMIS), and the Applied Cognition-Abilities and Applied Cognition-Concerns. If a patient screens positively, further evaluation with formal neuropsychological testing may be beneficial to further delineate the cognitive deficits and help guide treatment interventions. The most reliable way to document cognitive deficits is through neuropsychological testing, though this can be time-consuming and expensive, and access to providers may be limited.

Cognitive impairment due to cancer and cancer treatment requires medical and neuropsychological evaluation

Cognitive impairment secondary to cancer treatment is differentiated from other diagnoses based on a complete medical evaluation and psychiatric interview. Risk factors for cognitive impairment secondary to cancer treatment include a history of cognitive impairment, medical comorbidity (cardiovascular or neurovascular disease), cumulative exposure to cancer treatments (chemotherapy, immunotherapy, radiation), type and severity of malignancy, history of depression or anxiety, lower educational achievement, and advanced age. The underlying cause of cognitive impairment in patients with cancer has not been fully elucidated and is likely the result of multiple factors. These factors include genetic predisposition, oxidative stress and systemic inflammation, immune dysfunction, direct neurotoxic effects of cancer and cancer treatments causing accelerated aging of neuronal cells, and response to psychological stress triggering the hypothalamic-pituitary-adrenal axis. Additionally, patients diagnosed with any type of brain cancer have an elevated risk for cognitive impairment, which varies depending on the type and location of the cancer.

The treatment of cognitive impairment secondary to cancer treatments includes direct treatment of comorbid conditions, cognitive rehabilitation (including cognitive-behavioral interventions), exercise, and the possible addition of various stimulant medications. Cognitive remediation is an intervention that health psychologists can offer to address mild cognitive impairment associated with cancer treatment (Fernandes et al., 2019). This approach involves teaching the affected individual alternative strategies to supplement their usual cognitive processes, such as using a daily schedule or "sticky notes."

The goal of treatment for mild cognitive impairment is remission of symptoms; however, because of the unique nature of this syndrome, remission may not be achievable, and maximizing independent functioning and QoL becomes the goal. Symptoms may emerge at any point in the cancer continuum, and ongoing monitoring is required for early identification and intervention.

3.7   Substance Use Disorders (SUD)

According to DSM-5 (APA, 2013), a SUD is defined as a collection of symptoms and behaviors leading to clinically significant impairment caused by substance use. In general, these symptoms include a lack of control over substance use with frequent urges to use. Patients attempts to quit have been unsuccessful and they experience significant impairment in multiple domains of their life. Patients may continue to use the substance despite experiencing unwanted consequences. Patients will begin to require larger amounts of the substance to achieve intoxication and may experience physical or psychological withdrawal when they stop using the substance. The severity of the SUD is determined based on the number of symptoms present. There are 10 classes of drugs identified in SUDs: alcohol, caffeine, cannabis, hallucinogens (PCP and other hallucinogens), inhalants, opioids, sedatives/hypnotics/anxiolytics, stimulants (amphetamine, cocaine, and other stimulants), tobacco, and other/unknown substance. (For further reading on the specific diagnostic criteria, readers are encouraged to reference the DSM-5 directly.)

The incidence and prevalence of SUDs in the general population vary depending on many factors, and the same is true for patients with cancer. Data published on this topic suggest the possibility of lower rates of SUDs in this population than in the general population, although the studies were generally small and may have underreported the prevalence of SUDs (Holland, 2010). Patients with cancer may have a pre-existing SUD, involving tobacco or alcohol, that contributed to the development of their cancer. For these patients, treatment of the SUD may also improve their disease-specific outcomes. Patients with cancer can also develop SUDs because of substance use to cope with the negative physical and psychological symptoms of cancer.

Management of pain in cancer may present some unique challenges for patients as many are prescribed opioid medication in addition to nonopioid analgesics. Parallel to the increasing awareness and concern regarding the opioid epidemic, patients and medical providers struggle to minimize the risk of harm while also adequately treating pain. The vast majority of patients with cancer can safely be prescribed adequate doses of opioids for pain management and not develop an SUD; however, some patients do develop aberrant drug-related behaviors that may signify the onset of an SUD. Aberrant drug-related behaviors suggestive of an SUD include selling or forging prescriptions, stealing or borrowing other's medications, obtaining prescription drugs from nonmedical sources, and repeatedly taking medication in a way other than prescribed (Holland, 2010). Aberrant drug-related behaviors that are less suggestive of an SUD include complaining about uncontrolled pain and need for higher doses of medication, hoarding prescriptions in preparation for worsening pain, unapproved use of medication to treat symptoms other than pain, and report of altered states of consciousness not intended by the prescriber (Holland, 2010). It is important to pay attention to patients who may be misusing their prescription opioids to treat symptoms other than pain because this will suggest other interventions needed to help relieve distress. For example, patients may self-medicate with opioids to treat anxiety, insomnia, or psychological pain. Further investigation into the underlying cause of such symptoms and a follow-up with adaptive treatment planning may minimize inappropriate prescription drug use and lower the overall risk of an SUD.

SUDs are often included in the differential diagnosis for cognitive, mood, anxiety, trauma-related, or psychotic disorders. Depending on the disorder in question, there is variable incidence and prevalence of a comorbid SUD. It is beyond the scope of this book to go into the details of each individual SUD and the rates of other comorbid psychiatric disorders. The important point here is that all patients should complete periodic screening for substance use, and SUDs should remain in the differential diagnosis until they have been ruled out.

Treatment for SUDs often involves a combination of behavioral modification, self-help groups, and individual and group therapy. Medication-assisted therapy may also be recommended in the cases of alcohol, sedative, opioid, and tobacco use disorders. The goal for treatment varies depending on the patient's self-identified goals, the severity of use, medical complications secondary to use, the presence of withdrawal symptoms occurring with abrupt cessation, and the interpersonal/occupational/legal ramifications of current or future use. In many cases, the clinician recommends minimization or com-

Opioid medications can be safely prescribed to most patients with cancer without significant risk of developing a SUD

Not all aberrant drug-related behaviors are suggestive of an SUD

All patients should be screened for substance use

Treatment for SUDs involves a partnership between the clinician and the patient focused on the patient's goals

plete cessation of the relevant substance. Yet, the patient may have their own preferences about their current use and may not completely agree with recommendations to limit or stop use. In these instances, motivational interviewing is an evidence-based approach to evaluate the patient's interest in addressing the problem and to promote the consideration of behavior change (Smedslund et al. 2011).

3.8   Vulnerable Populations

Lower socioeconomic status has been associated with higher rates of distress primarily driven by financial distress (Meeker et al., 2016). Financial difficulties is often exacerbated because of limitations on a patient's ability to work while going through treatment. Many individuals do not have eligibility for short or long-term disability benefits through their employer; therefore, the inability to work can drastically reduce income, causing problems with housing, utilities, food, and transportation.

Lower socioeconomic status, rural setting, and pre-existing psychiatric diagnosis contribute to health disparities

Patients with cancer living in rural settings have greater disparities in the incidence of cancer, and in access to cancer diagnostics and cancer treatment, all of which likely explain poorer rates of survival (Atkins et al., 2017; Paskett et al., 2020). These disparities can arise because of a lack of access to the healthcare system or greater distance of travel to obtain subspecialty screening and treatment. Providing distress assessment and psychosocial treatments via telehealth (including telephone-based services) can reduce barriers to needed support. Telehealth became more widely available with the COVID-19 pandemic.

Historically, patients with pre-existing psychiatric diagnoses have had worse cancer outcomes

Individuals with pre-existing psychiatric diagnoses have worse overall survival and worse prognosis in the context of cancer, due in part to their decreased likelihood of getting timely cancer care consistent with established clinical guidelines (Kisely et al., 2013; Paredes et al., 2021). In fact, those diagnosed with schizophrenia have increased mortality from breast, colorectal, and lung cancer (Kisely et al., 2013). The intake interview should include questions about history of mental-health diagnoses or active mental-health symptoms. When possible, patients with such a history can be referred to specialty care. Some settings may present scant resources for mental-health treatment, in which case distress screening proves less useful; however, with increasing awareness of the problems that patients with cancer face, more resources are becoming available.

Adolescents and Young Adults (AYAs)

The psychosocial needs of AYAs are often fundamentally different from those of older patients and pediatric patients. The combination of typical developmental transitions in early adulthood and the physical and emotional impact of cancer can place AYAs at heightened risk for cancer-related distress. In particular, processes of separation/individuation can be disrupted in families dealing with cancer in an adolescent or young adult. AYA patients can also experience significantly longer periods of survivorship than other groups, again pointing to the need for psychosocial support and intervention across the

AYAs are confronted with unique issues because of their developmental stage and their extended cancer survivorship

care continuum. Treatment of distress among AYAs with cancer should incorporate evaluation of concerns across several potential domains: health behaviors, peer relations, fertility and family planning, family dynamics, financial, career/education, trust in healthcare, emotions, body image, and self-esteem (Nass et al., 2015).

4

Treatment

More frequent screening and identification of needs among cancer patients, families, and caregivers have heightened the need for access to psychosocial care, and allied health professionals are now considered to be important members of cancer-care teams. Treatment of cancer-related distress is multimodal and can be delivered by several potential team members via multiple models of care.

This chapter provides an overview of evidence-based psychotherapies that are effective for minimizing distress, enhancing coping, and improving QoL, as well as an overview of commonly prescribed psychiatric medications for the management of psychiatric comorbidities. While not reviewed in this book, other components of integrative medicine, such as acupuncture, massage, nutritional counseling, spiritual counseling or pastoral care, and palliative care, can all be useful approaches to managing a variety of cancer-related physical and psychiatric symptoms. As in patients without cancer, patients with cancer often benefit from combined modalities, such as combined antidepressant and cognitive behavioral therapy (CBT) for patients with comorbid cancer and depression. These interventions can be delivered via a variety of service models, including consultative services that are directly linked to distress screening, integrated or co-located care, and collaborative care.

Distress screening (previously described) is most effective when integrated into standard oncologic care and can assist with identifying psychosocial needs among cancer patients. One component of the CoC requirements for distress screening is to link patients with needed psychosocial services onsite or through referral to outside agencies. In its most basic form, this model of care might include a resource list of internal hospital providers or local or national cancer support resources, which can be provided to patients when concerns are identified. Increasingly, high-volume cancer centers are capitalizing on the electronic medical records (EMRs) to conduct frequent, systematic distress screening, which then generates timely notifications to relevant allied healthcare professionals who connect with patients to further evaluate needs, potentially provide brief psychotherapeutic intervention, and link the patient to needed services. This type of care model may also include mental-health professionals who are available by page for managing acute distress, or who work in a clinic for a particular disease site or disease stage, such as a comprehensive breast cancer clinic or survivorship clinic.

Integrated, or co-located care refers to supportive oncology services that are offered to patients within a cancer center by a multitude of specialists. For example, a psychologist, psychiatrist, or social worker may be employed by a cancer center and available to see patients at various stages of the cancer care continuum. Supportive services are considered an important part of the patient's comprehensive cancer treatment and serve to ensure cancer care is patient-centered and holistic. Any of the treatments described in this chapter may be delivered in an integrated care setting.

Lastly, collaborative care is a patient-centered, integrated medical-behavioral model for delivering psychiatric care to patients in medical environments. This model of care is described in greater detail later in this chapter.

Interventions can be delivered at any point across the cancer continuum, and modified to address the unique presenting concerns at each stage. According to the Institute of Medicine (2013), palliative and psychosocial care for patients and caregivers/families should span the cancer continuum from diagnosis through end-of-life, and should account for the fact that patients may enter the continuum at any stage and may not progress sequentially (see Figure 1).

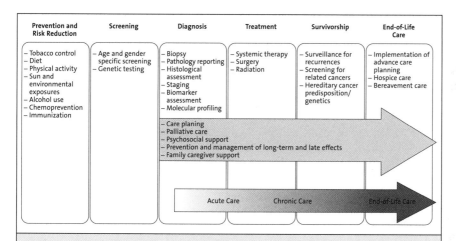

Figure 1
The Institute of Medicine's conceptualization of the cancer care continuum from diagnosis through end-of-life care (2013, p. 4). © National Academy of Sciences. Reprinted with permission.

4.1   Methods of Treatment

4.1.1   Psychotherapy

Several psychotherapeutic interventions have been utilized and studied among a variety of cancer populations. Specific cancer topics that arise in therapy may include the impact of physical illness, beliefs and expectations about the illness (how the disease will progress, fear of recurrence), concerns about current and future ability to cope, loss of control, uncertainty, difficulty accepting help and role changes, and acceptance of cancer and cancer-related changes, and end-of-life concerns. Below we review the most commonly used psychotherapies.

Cognitive Behavioral Therapy

Cognitive behavioral therapy (CBT) is considered an effective first-line treatment for many psychiatric conditions in the general population. CBT generally has three components: self-monitoring, behavior change (behavioral activation, exposure-based techniques, relaxation strategies, modification of maladaptive behaviors), and cognitive restructuring of both automatic distorted thoughts and core beliefs about oneself, others, and the world. Each of these components has been modified and validated for a multitude of conditions, including depression, anxiety, insomnia, and chronic pain. Traditional CBT interventions are used in cancer populations for the treatment of both comorbid mood and anxiety disorders as well as for cancer symptoms and treatment-related side effects (Akechi et al., 2008; Osborn et al., 2006). CBT is also effective for improving QoL in cancer patients (Getu et al., 2020).

In the case of depression and anxiety, CBT in cancer populations may resemble CBT for patients without cancer, with potential differences lying in the content of patients' thoughts and associated maladaptive behaviors, and with an additional focus on the relationship between thoughts, emotions, behaviors, and the physical impact of the disease. There is often a particular focus on stress management and problem-solving (Antoni et al., 2009), and CBT in cancer tends to focus more heavily on the development of active coping strategies (over avoidant or passive coping) than on challenging cognitions. Worry management is often a useful focus given the varied types of worries associated with cancer (e.g., anticipations of scans and results, worry about the effectiveness of treatment, fear of cancer recurrence). It may be more difficult to discern catastrophizing in the context of a cancer diagnosis, particularly with more advanced stages of the disease. In some situations, it can be helpful to get a medical perspective on how well the patient's perception of their prognosis matches with the perspective of the medical team, as there can be mismatches in both directions (patients may see the prognosis as worse or better than the physician). Behavioral activation can be more difficult in the cancer setting if fatigue is an issue.

CBT is also well established in the treatment of cancer symptoms and treatment side effects. For example, there are established protocols for the treatment of insomnia (Johnson et al., 2016; Ma et al., 2021), pain (Ehde et al., 2014), and fatigue (Hilfiker et al., 2018) – common side effects in the person with cancer. Also, CBT can be very effective in the management of anticipatory nausea (Hagmann et al., 2018).

Mindfulness Interventions

Mindfulness-based approaches have been utilized in cancer care to support patients to achieve self-regulation, present moment awareness, and acceptance of experience without judgment. Several reviews document benefits of mindfulness-based interventions including decreased distress, improved sleep, reduced fatigue, improved mood (anxiety, depression), and a heightened sense of well-being and QoL (Cillessen et al., 2019; Xunlin et al., 2020). Mindfulness is thought to be particularly appropriate for the non-problem-focused issues that can arise for patients with cancer, such as coping with loss of control, uncertainty, loss and grief (versus issues such as promoting adherence to complex medication regimens). Using mindfulness approaches, patients can learn to accept and even embrace change and uncertainty by allowing themselves to live more fully in the present moment. There are several mindfulness-based approaches specifically for patients with cancer, perhaps most notably Mindfulness-Based Cancer Recovery (MBCR), developed by Linda Carlson and Michael Speca (2011) and Mindfulness-Based Cognitive Therapy (MBCT; Park et al., 2020). MBCR is an 8-week program that includes body awareness exercises, meditation, and gentle yoga, practiced both in class and through daily home practice. MBCT is a similar 8-week program, with more focus on the relationship between mood, cognition, and overall functioning.

Acceptance and Commitment Therapy

Acceptance and commitment therapy (ACT) is a third-wave CBT that includes a variety of strategies aimed at modifying patients' relationships with their thoughts and feelings so that they can experience painful internal experiences without being dominated by them. Patients work to clarify their values and commit to engaging in value-consistent activities, rather than choosing behaviors that attempt to control or reduce painful thoughts, emotions, and sensations. Acceptance strategies, including cognitive defusion and mindfulness techniques, are also utilized to help patients cope effectively with distressing physical symptoms. Several randomized and controlled outcome studies have yielded positive findings for ACT in the context of chronic health conditions, including improved mood and QoL among cancer patients (Feros et al., 2013; González-Fernández & Fernández-Rodríguez, 2019; Hulbert-Williams et al., 2015).

ACT has six primary components that form the hexaflex model (Hayes, Strosahl, & Wilson, 1999) (see Figure 2). Each component can be applied

Acceptance and commitment therapy is a third-wave cognitive-behavioral therapy that emphasizes acceptance of thoughts and circumstances and commitment to values-based action

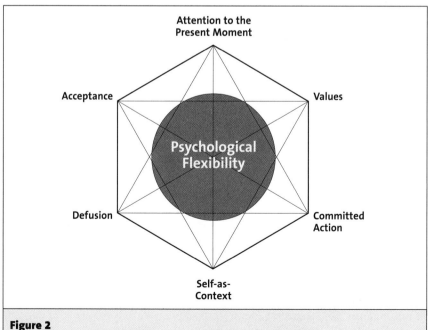

Figure 2
The Hexaflex Model. © Steven C. Hayes. Used with permission.

to the experience of patients with cancer. Patients learn to take a stance of openness toward their internal and external experiences, whether perceived as good or bad (present moment awareness, acceptance). They practice reducing their attachment to the content of their cognitions to weaken the impact those cognitions have on mood and behavior (cognitive defusion). For example, a person with a history of smoking who has developed cancer may ruminate on thoughts of self-blame, accordingly feel distress, and consequently exhibit less active involvement with care. Defusing those thoughts offers the patient space to choose more effective behaviors, such as taking an active role in treatment (coming on time to appointments, exercising, making healthy diet changes, etc.). ACT can be useful for helping patients to explore identity issues, such as distinguishing between "being a cancer patient" and "being a person who has cancer" (self-as-context). Lastly, patients participating in ACT in the context of cancer care can explore shifts in their values as a result of cancer experiences and enhance commitment to living their life in a manner consistent with their values (committed action).

Meaning-Centered Psychotherapy

Meaning-centered psychotherapy focuses on helping individuals find meaning and purpose as they face advanced cancer

Meaning-centered psychotherapy (MCP) is grounded in the works of Victor Frankl and specifically tailored to patients with advanced cancer. MCP utilizes didactics, reflection, clarification, exploration, and experiential exercises to help patients with advanced cancer discover meaning, peace, and purpose as they face increasing limitations associated with disease progression. The efficacy of MCP has been demonstrated in both individual and group formats, with improved QoL and spiritual well-being, decreased anxiety, and decreased desire for hastened death (Breitbart et al., 2010; Breitbart et al., 2018). Components of the intervention include exploring a patient's cancer story, understanding the patient's sense of identity and the impact of cancer on their identity, and exploring multiple sources of meaning (historical, attitudinal, creative, and experiential). Participants also work on a Legacy Project, which includes examination of their legacy as reflected in their past and lived in the present. This legacy work is therapeutic for the patient and can be passed on to loved ones if the patient chooses.

Dignity Therapy

Dignity therapy is an intervention for individuals at the end of life and focuses on creation of a legacy document

Dignity therapy is a brief, focused intervention developed by Harvey Chochinov for individuals at the end of life (Chochinov et al., 2005). Therapists conduct a life review with the individual and develop a legacy document capturing the essence of the individual and their life experience. The legacy document is created through a focused interview by the therapist and subsequent transcription of the interview. An important step is the individual receiving and reviewing the document before it is passed on to family members. This intervention is associated with decreased anxiety and depression in participants (Martínez et al., 2017).

Supportive Psychotherapy

Many patients with cancer benefit from supportive psychotherapy, particularly when they do not meet the criteria for a comorbid psychiatric diagnosis. Supportive psychotherapy consists of therapeutic interventions that aim to help patients manage distressing emotions or physical experiences, reinforce pre-existing coping strengths, and promote the development of new adaptive coping strategies. Specific interventions may include: helping to process and clarify complex or upsetting information about the disease, supporting problem-solving, flexibly using a range of strategies to support adaptive coping, offering a safe supportive space for emotional processing and expression, normalizing and validating the patient's experience, supporting the patient's family, linking to resources, and serving as a liaison with the primary medical team. Supportive psychotherapy can be delivered across all treatment models and care settings and is most beneficial when the provider has a sound knowledge of cancer and the unique experiences of patients with cancer.

Supportive psychotherapy may help to manage distressing experiences, reinforce coping strengths, and develop coping strategies

4.1.2   Groups and Other Approaches

Support Groups

Support groups are a common supportive intervention among cancer populations and focus on a combination of psychoeducation and peer support to facilitate coping and living with cancer. Groups are typically facilitated by an allied health professional, who can help by keeping the group on the topic. Support groups offer a unique sense of community, particularly in contrast to the common experience of feeling isolated and misunderstood in noncancer communities. Patients have reported heightened empowerment and agency because of participation in support groups as well as appreciation for the safe space for exploring emotional issues, which can reduce the burden on outside supports (Ussher et al., 2006). Groups aim to create a space for peer support, emotional expression and validation, exploration and demystification of end-of-life issues; and to facilitate the sharing of information, resources, and coping strategies. Support groups can focus on specific cancer types (e.g., breast, prostate), demographic variables (e.g., young adults), or phase of care (e.g., newly diagnosed, survivorship, end of life).

Support groups provide psychoeducation, peer support, and exposure to new resources or strategies

Grief Therapy

Elisabeth Kubler-Ross changed the public discourse about grief when she published her work on the stages of grief (Kübler-Ross, 1969). She proposed five stages in response to a loss: denial, anger, bargaining, depression, and acceptance. While all of these are common reactions to death or impending death, her model has been interpreted to mean that these are sequential stages a grieving person goes through – and that once you get to acceptance, your grief is resolved. As more research has been done in the area, it has become clear that the five stages can happen in any order, that not everyone experiences every stage, and that any particular stage can be experienced multiple times.

Grief therapy can be used to address anticipatory grief for patients with a terminal disease or to support family caregivers in anticipation of or in follow-up to their loved one's death. The goal of grief therapy is not to bring resolution to an individual's grief, but instead to help them find a state that allows them to move forward in life with their grief. The intervention may include normalizing and validating the person's experience of loss and grief. Unfortunately, it is not unusual for well-meaning friends or acquaintances to

Grief therapy can be utilized to address losses associated with cancer, anticipatory grief, and bereavement

offer well-meaning expressions, like "It's for the best" or "God needed an angel" or "It's time to get on with your life." Given the unhelpful reactions and advice of others, grief therapy sometimes needs to include a focus on strategizing how to manage the comments and behavior of others. Finally, grief therapy may incorporate an ACT-type focus on values-based living, helping the grieving individual to identify future-oriented goals consistent with their values.

Interventions for Partners, Families, and Caregivers

The previously reviewed psychotherapies can be delivered not only to patients but also to caregivers and family members, with or without the patient present. Caregivers can experience both physical and emotional demands because of caregiving responsibilities, many of which can strain their personal time, social roles, financial resources, and health. Accordingly, caregivers experience a wide range of psychological complications (e.g., fear, depression, anxiety, guilt, anticipatory grief), physical complications (e.g., sleep difficulties, poor immune functioning, lack of health service utilization, decrease in healthy lifestyle behaviors), and psychosocial challenges (e.g., disruptions in work or income; Applebaum & Breitbart, 2013). Similarly, couples often experience adjustment-related difficulties such as communication challenges and heightened conflict, loss of intimacy, loss of mutual support, concerns about parenting, and shifts in typical family roles and responsibilities (Baik & Adams, 2011). Supporting couples and caregivers with psychosocial interventions is a vital part of promoting the health and success of the patient with cancer.

> Caregivers experience physical and emotional challenges as they support someone with cancer

4.1.3   Medications

Psychotropic medications are commonly prescribed in the oncology setting to treat psychiatric disorders, symptoms related to cancer, and the side effects of cancer treatment. Here, we provide a brief overview of many of the commonly prescribed medications separated by drug class.

Antidepressants

Antidepressants are commonly prescribed for depression and anxiety disorders that occur during any stage of the cancer continuum. The most common agents are listed in Table 2 below.

Antidepressants have varied mechanisms of action. The medications are separated, based on common nomenclature, into four distinct categories: selective serotonin reuptake inhibitors (SSRIs), serotonin and norepinephrine reuptake inhibitors (SNRIs), atypical antidepressants, and tricyclic antidepressants (TCAs). All antidepressants carry a black-box warning label for suicidal ideation in patients under 25 years. Common side effects of these medications are listed in the table. Sometimes these "side effects" can be the goal when targeting specific symptoms as noted in the off-label/adjunctive use column. Special attention should be paid to all medications regarding the potential for interactions with other prescribed and over-the-counter medications as well as herbal and nutritional supplements.

> Some side effects of antidepressants may be leveraged to treat unwanted symptoms of cancer and cancer treatment

Table 2
Commonly Prescribed Antidepressants for Patients With Cancer

Medication class	Medication name (trade name)	Typical dose range (mg/day)	Indications	Off-label/adjunctive uses	Common possible side effects
Selective serotonin reuptake inhibitors (SSRIs)	Citalopram (Celexa)	10–40	Depressive disorders, anxiety disorders, PTSD	None	Headache, gastrointestinal distress, sexual dysfunction
	Escitalopram (Lexapro)	2.5–20			Headache, gastrointestinal distress, sexual dysfunction
	Fluoxetine (Prozac)	10–80			Headache, gastrointestinal distress, sexual dysfunction, weight gain, transient increase in anxiety
	Paroxetine (Paxil)	5–60			Headache, gastrointestinal distress, sexual dysfunction, sedation, dry mouth, dizziness, discontinuation syndrome
	Sertraline (Zoloft)	25–250			Headache, gastrointestinal distress, sexual dysfunction
Selective norepinephrine reuptake inhibitors (SNRIs)	Duloxetine (Cymbalta)	30–120	Depressive disorders, anxiety disorders, PTSD	Neuropathic pain, hot flashes	Gastrointestinal distress, dizziness, sexual dysfunction, blurred vision
	Venlafaxine (Effexor)	37.5–300			Gastrointestinal distress, sexual dysfunction, small increase in blood pressure, discontinuation syndrome
	Desvenlafaxine (Pristiq)	25–50			Gastrointestinal distress, dizziness, headache, blurred vision

Table 2. Continued

Medication class	Medication name (trade name)	Typical dose range (mg/day)	Indications	Off-label/adjunctive uses	Common possible side effects
Atypical antidepressants	Bupropion (Wellbutrin)	75–450	Depressive disorders	Attention, focus, energy, motivation; few sexual side effects	Lower seizure threshold, headache, nausea
	Mirtazapine (Remeron)	7.5–45	Depressive disorders	Insomnia, anorexia/cachexia, reduced anxiety	Dry mouth, sedation, weight gain
	Trazodone (Desyrel)	25–300	Depressive disorders	Insomnia, agitation	Highly sedating, orthostatic hypotension, sexual dysfunction
Tricyclic antidepressants (TCAs)	Amitriptyline (Elavil)	25–150	Major depressive disorder, anxiety disorders	Insomnia, neuropathic pain and other pain syndromes, migraine prevention	Sedation, GI upset, orthostatic hypotension, QT prolongation, urinary retention, constipation
	Nortriptyline (Pamelor)	25–150	Major depressive disorders	Neuropathic pain and other pain syndromes, migraine prevention	Sedation, GI upset, orthostatic hypotension, QT prolongation, urinary retention, constipation
	Clomipramine (Anafranil)	25–250	Obsessive compulsive disorder, major depressive disorder		Sedation, GI upset, orthostatic hypotension, QT prolongation, urinary retention, constipation

Benzodiazepines

Benzodiazepines are rapid-acting medications that specifically target symptoms related to anxiety that can occur during any stage of the cancer continuum. These medications are most effective for severe and/or acute anxiety, panic, anxiety that interferes with sleep, and anxiety that causes nausea or vomiting. Ideally, these medications are prescribed in a time-limited fashion until other interventions have provided long-lasting relief of symptoms.

All benzodiazepines carry a risk of tolerance as well as physiological and psychological dependence. After long-term use, immediate cessation of benzodiazepines can lead to withdrawal, which can be severe and potentially life-threatening. Symptoms of withdrawal include anxiety, irritability, agitation, altered mental status, tachycardia, hypertension, and seizures. Treatment for withdrawal includes resuming the benzodiazepine. If the intention of treatment shifts to discontinuing a benzodiazepine, then a slow, planned taper should be implemented. These medications can also be used to treat alcohol withdrawal. The mechanism of action of these medications occurs via action at the gamma-amino butyric acid receptor leading to inhibition of the central nervous system and anxiolysis. Each of the medications has a unique duration of effect that can be utilized to target specific presentations of anxiety (see Table 3).

Avoid abrupt cessation of benzodiazepines to prevent a potentially dangerous withdrawal syndrome

Antipsychotics

Antipsychotics are commonly prescribed for primary psychotic disorders including schizophrenia and schizoaffective disorders. They exhibit utility in the treatment of bipolar disorder when used in addition to mood stabilizers. They can also be useful in the treatment of severe agitation that occurs in the setting of hyperactive delirium. Additionally, they have demonstrated effectiveness in the treatment of major depressive disorder when used in combination with other antidepressants. When few clinical alternatives exist, they can be utilized in low doses for the treatment of anxiety symptoms and disorders; however, this should be done only when all other options for treatment have been evaluated. All antipsychotics carry the black-box warning concerning early death in elderly patients with dementia. All antipsychotics may cause extrapyramidal symptoms (akathisia, parkinsonism, acute dystonia) or tardive dyskinesia. Nearly all antipsychotics can lead to a prolongation of the QT interval of the cardiac cycle, which in turn can lead to life-threatening cardiac arrhythmia in rare instances. The degree to which the QT segment is prolonged is often determined by multiple factors including comorbid medical problems, polypharmacy, and total antipsychotic dose. This topic is discussed further in the section on drug–drug interactions.

Antipsychotics can offer clinical benefit beyond the treatment of psychotic disorders

Antipsychotics can be separated into two different categories, first-generation (typical antipsychotics) and second-generation (atypical antipsychotics). There is some overlap in the mechanism of action of these two classes. However, first-generation/typical antipsychotics primarily exert their effects via a blockade of the dopamine receptor, specifically the D2 receptor; second-generation/atypical antipsychotics exert their effects primarily via a blockade of the serotonin receptor, specifically the 5HT-2a receptor, and blockade of the D2 receptor, albeit less than the first-generation antipsychotics. The side effect profile of each medication varies. The most common side effects are listed in Table 4.

Table 3
List of Commonly Prescribed Benzodiazepines

Medication class	Medication name (trade name)	Typical dose range (mg/day)	Indications	Off-label use	Side effects
Benzodiazepine anxiolytics	Alprazolam (Xanax)	0.125–2	Anxiety disorders		Short-acting, rebound anxiety, sedation, dizziness, loss of balance, memory problems
	Clonazepam (Klonopin)	0.25–4			Sedation, dizziness, loss of balance, memory problems
	Diazepam (Valium)	1–45		Muscle relaxant	Sedation, dizziness, loss of balance, memory problems
	Lorazepam (Ativan)	0.25–6		Nausea	Sedation, dizziness, loss of balance, memory problems

Table 4
List of Commonly Prescribed Antipsychotics

Medication class	Medication name (trade name)	Typical dose range (mg/day)	Indication	Off-label use	Side effects
Antipsychotics	Haloperidol (Haldol) first generation	0.25–20	Psychosis	Severe anxiety, agitation associated with delirium, nausea, and vomiting	Extrapyramidal symptoms, sedation, risk for cardiac arrhythmia as dose increases, orthostatic hypotension
	Aripiprazole (Abilify)	2–30	Psychosis, acute mania, treatment of resistant mood disorders	Less sedating than other similar medications	Metabolic syndrome, orthostatic hypotension
	Olanzapine (Zyprexa)	2.5–20	Psychosis, acute mania, treatment of resistant mood disorders	Severe anxiety, agitation associated with delirium, nausea, and vomiting	Metabolic syndrome, orthostatic hypotension, sedation, constipation
	Quetiapine (Seroquel)	12–5–800	Psychosis, acute Mania, treatment of resistant mood disorders	Severe anxiety, agitation associated with delirium	Metabolic syndrome, orthostatic hypotension, sedation
	Risperidone (Risperdal)	0.25–8	Psychosis, acute mania	Severe anxiety, agitation associated with delirium	Metabolic syndrome, orthostatic hypotension, sedation, constipation
	Ziprasidone (Geodon)	20–160	Psychosis, acute mania	Agitation associated with delirium	Metabolic syndrome, orthostatic hypotension, sedation, bradycardia

Stimulants

Stimulants are often prescribed for short-term relief of cancer related symptoms

Stimulants include medications in the amphetamine and amphetamine-like classes. Stimulants are most commonly prescribed for the treatment of attention-deficit hyperactivity disorder. In patients with cancer, stimulants may be prescribed off-label to treat cognitive deficits, fatigue, anhedonia, apathy, or demoralization that can occur at any time in the cancer continuum. Stimulants are sometimes prescribed in addition to other medications as an adjunctive treatment for major depressive disorder. The benefits of these medications may be seen immediately and typically wear off when the medication is discontinued. Although stimulants may be associated with reduced appetite, at low doses they may paradoxically increase appetite in this patient population. The mechanism of action includes increasing dopamine release as well as the prevention of dopamine reuptake. All stimulants have a small risk of tolerance, dependence, and irritability. Modafinil is a stimulant-like medication that has a unique and not fully understood mechanism of action, which likely involves the dopamine, norepinephrine, and histamine systems (see Table 5).

Hypnotics

Hypnotic use should be time-limited and based on situational factors that are expected to resolve

Hypnotics are a class of medications specifically designed to treat insomnia. Like the benzodiazepines mentioned before, hypnotics exert their mechanism of action on the gamma-amino butyric acid system leading to sedation via reduced central nervous system activation. They can be effective medications for the short-term management of early and middle insomnia; however, the American College of Physicians recommends psychotherapy as the first line of treatment for patients with chronic sleep difficulties (Qaseem, 2016). Data suggest that cognitive behavioral therapy of insomnia (CBT-I) has a superior benefit over hypnotics for treating insomnia in patients with cancer (Kripke, 2016). Frequent use of hypnotics often leads to tolerance and reduction in the effectiveness of the medication. While these medications are rarely abused, dependence is possible. Hypnotics are best used intermittently and over short durations to assist in the treatment of insomnia until an underlying cause of insomnia can be identified and treated. The use of hypnotics may also contribute to daytime sedation and impaired cognition. Additionally, the use of these medications may lead to parasomnias such as sleepeating or sleepwalking (see Table 6).

Anticonvulsants/Mood Stabilizers

Anticonvulsants and mood stabilizers are a broad category of medications for the treatment of seizure disorders, bipolar disorder, and pain. Each medication in this group has a unique mechanism of action. In patients with cancer, these medications are most often used for the management of neuropathic pain or mood stabilization for comorbid bipolar disorder. Valproic acid can be used for the management of agitation in delirium or irritability and mood lability in brain cancers. The common side effects of these medications are included in Table 7.

Table 5
List of Commonly Prescribed Stimulants

Medication class	Medication name (trade name)	Typical dose range (mg/day)	Indications	Off-label use	Side effects
Amphetamine-based stimulants	Amphetamine/dextroamphetamine		Attention deficit hyperactivity disorder	Cognitive impairment secondary to cancer treatment, severe fatigue, apathy, and demoralization	Insomnia, anxiety, appetite suppression, tachycardia
	Adderall	2.5–40			
	Adderall CR	5–20	Attention deficit hyperactivity disorder	Cognitive impairment secondary to cancer treatment, severe fatigue, apathy, and demoralization	Insomnia, anxiety, appetite suppression, tachycardia
Nonamphetamine-based stimulants	Methylphenidate (Concerta, Ritalin, Focalin)	Concerta – 18–72 Ritalin – 5–60 Focalin – 1.25–20	Attention deficit hyperactivity disorder	Cognitive impairment secondary to cancer treatment, severe fatigue, apathy, and demoralization	Insomnia, anxiety, appetite suppression, tachycardia
	Modafinil (Provigil)	50–200	Narcolepsy, obstructive sleep apnea, shiftwork sleep disorder	Cognitive impairment secondary to cancer treatment, severe fatigue, apathy, and demoralization	Insomnia, headache, nausea, diarrhea, anxiety

Table 6
List of Commonly Prescribed Hypnotics

Medication class	Medication name (trade name)	Typical dose range (mg/day)	Indications	Off-label use	Side effects
Hypnotics	Eszopiclone (Lunesta)	1–3	Insomnia		Headache, hallucinations, dizziness
	Zolpidem (Ambien)	2.5–10	Insomnia		Headache, hallucinations, dizziness, sleep-eating, other parasomnias

Table 7
List of Commonly Prescribed Mood Stabilizers and Anticonvulsants

Medication class	Medication name (trade name)	Typical dose range (mg/day)	Indications	Off-label use	Side effects
Anticonvulsants/mood stabilizers	Gabapentin (Neurontin)	100–2700	Neuropathic pain	Anxiety	Sedation, dizziness
	Pregabalin (Lyrica)	50–300	Neuropathic pain	Anxiety	Sedation, dizziness
	Lamotrigine (Lamictal)	25–200	Bipolar disorder, epilepsy and related seizure disorders		Nausea, rare life-threatening skin rash (Stevens-Johnson syndrome), headache
	Valproic acid (Depakote, Depakene)	250–2500	Bipolar disorder, epilepsy, and related seizure disorder	Agitation and irritability associated with brain injury	Sedation, hepatotoxicity, hyperammonemia, weight gain, bone marrow suppression

Drug–Drug Interactions

As cancer treatment continues to evolve, new medications and immunotherapies become available every year. Physicians must be mindful of the potential for drug-drug interactions when prescribing any medication to a patient receiving treatment for cancer. Because of the complexity of medical treatment and the many patients who require multiple medications, it can be helpful to involve a pharmacist as a member of the multidisciplinary team. Additionally, some screening programs exist that help to identify potential drug–drug interactions. A quick internet search reveals multiple websites that can be utilized to screen the patient's medications for possible drug interactions. These include pharmacy, university, and independent company websites. We do not recommend any single resource and ultimately recommend consulting the patient's physicians and pharmacist if any concerns arise.

The list of all potential medication interactions is exhaustive. Here, we attempt to describe some common concepts and drug-drug interactions that will be instructive to clinicians and physicians when treating patients with cancer.

Many medications prescribed to treat pain, anxiety, insomnia, and nausea/vomiting cause sedation as a side effect. It is not uncommon for patients to receive multiple prescriptions for these medications at any given time. A common example is a patient taking opioids for pain management, gabapentin or pregabalin for neuropathic pain, and benzodiazepines for anxiety, nausea, or insomnia. Combinations of multiple sedating medications can become dangerous because of the additive sedating effect these medications have on each other. When these medications are used in combination, patients can experience profound sedation, lethargy, confusion or cognitive impairment, loss of coordination, increased risk of falls, altered mental status and delirium, and respiratory depression. At times these symptoms are dangerous and potentially life-threatening. No absolute contraindication exists for combining multiple sedating medications, and often they are necessary to relieve suffering. Nevertheless, close observation, use of the lowest possible dose to achieve the therapeutic benefit, and discontinuing medication when no longer indicated are all necessary practices to minimize the risk of harm to the patient.

Another common example of drug-drug interactions is the additive effect medications can have on the QT interval of the cardiac conduction cycle. The QT interval represents the amount of time it takes for the ventricles of the heart to contract and relax. This is visually represented on an electrocardiogram, which measures the electrical conduction through the heart. The QTc is a calculation of the QT interval with correction for the patient's heartrate. When this interval becomes prolonged for any reason, the patient is at higher risk of cardiac arrhythmia, which may become life-threatening. Numerous medications, including some psychiatric medications, can lead to prolongation of this interval. For a brief overview of common psychiatric medications known to increase the QT interval, please refer to Table 8 below. For a list of other common medications known to impact the QT interval, please refer to Table 9 below. When any of these medications are used in combination, the impact on the QT interval is multiplied, further increasing the risk for arrhythmia. It is common for patients with cancer to be prescribed multiple medications that can prolong the QT interval. For example, many patients with cancer are pre-

Avoidance of drug–drug interactions requires vigilant surveillance by all members of the multidisciplinary team

Drug–drug interactions are due to additive side effects or alterations of drug metabolism

scribed antiemetic medications to manage the side effects of chemotherapy, antibiotics to treat infections while the patient is immunocompromised, and psychiatric medications to manage psychiatric symptoms. Patients on combination therapy should undergo regular monitoring with an electrocardiogram to identify instances of prolonged QT interval. If the QTc is prolonged, follow-up should include modification of the medication regimen to reduce the risk of arrhythmia. For a more in-depth review of this topic, please refer to the review article by Xiong et al. (2020).

Table 8
Impact of Common Psychiatric Medications of QT Interval

Drug class	Drug name	Effect on QT interval (in ms)
Antipsychotic	Haloperidol intravenous	+16
	Haloperidol intramuscular or oral	+4–9
	Ziprasidone	+16
	Quetiapine	+15
	Risperidone	+10
	Olanzapine	+6
	Paliperidone	+4
	Aripiprazole	-4
Antidepressant	Citalopram	+10–20
	Escitalopram	+5–11
	Amitriptyline	+1–20
	Trazodone	-4–7

Adapted from Xiong et al., 2020.

Many medications are metabolized through the liver via the cytochrome P450 (CYP 450) enzymes. These enzymes exist in all humans, yet there are genetic differences in the level of activity for any given subset of enzymes within this system. Additionally, some medications can act as inducers of these enzymes, meaning they increase the processing speed of the enzyme, leading to a more rapid metabolism of other medications that are normally broken down by that enzyme. This can be problematic when the anticancer medication is processed too quickly and rendered less effective in treating the patient's cancer. One example of this type of drug-drug interaction would be the combination of modafinil, a stimulant-like medication, and exemestane, an aromatase inhibitor used in the treatment of specific types of breast cancer. When modafinil is given to a patient taking exemestane, modafinil induces the activity of the CYP 450 3A4 subtype, leading to more rapid metabolism of exemestane and reduced drug effectiveness.

Table 9
List of Common Medications Known to Prolong QTc

Drug class	Drug name
Antiarrhythmic	Amiodarone
	Sotalol
Antibiotic	Ciprofloxacin
	Levofloxacin
	Azithromycin
	Clarithromycin
	Erythromycin
Antifungal	Fluconazole
	Ketoconazole
	Itraconazole
Opioid	Methadone
Antiemetic	Ondansetron
	Metoclopramide
	Prochlorperazine
	Promethazine
Antimigraine	Sumatriptan

Some medications act as inhibitors of these enzymes, meaning they slow the processing speed of the enzyme, which may cause excessive or toxic levels of medications to accrue. This in turn may cause a patient to experience adverse side effects of certain medications because the medications linger in their system longer than they should. Additionally, some medications require metabolism by the CYP 450 system to go from an inactive form of the drug to an active form of the drug. If the enzyme responsible for this conversion is inhibited, the process of going from an inactive drug to an active drug is slowed, which can result in a subtherapeutic treatment effect, leaving the patient at risk for a poorer response to treatment. One classic example of this phenomenon is the combination of tamoxifen, a selective estrogen receptor modulator used to prevent the recurrence of specific types of breast cancer, and medications for depression that inhibit the CYP 450 subset of enzymes labeled as 2D6. Antidepressants that strongly inhibit the CYP 450 2D6 activity include fluoxetine, paroxetine, and duloxetine; antidepressants that moderately inhibit the enzyme activity include citalopram, escitalopram, and sertraline. If tamoxifen is combined with any of these medications, it does not get as readily converted into an active form, increasing the risk of breast

Drug–drug interactions can have serious consequences for cancer treatment and require close monitoring

cancer recurrence. Often, the first-line treatment for depression for a patient taking tamoxifen is venlafaxine because it does not have this same interaction. The same phenomenon described above is observed as well with the anticancer drugs vinblastine and doxorubicin in combination with other CYP450 2D6 inhibitors.

Off Label Use

Several of the medications previously described have off-label uses that can be particularly helpful in managing common symptoms of cancer and side effects of treatment. These off-label uses can be found in a column in each of the medication tables. This is not an exhaustive list; however, it is meant to outline some of the most common off-label uses for psychiatric medications. For example, mirtazapine is often used to stimulate appetite and to facilitate sleep. Trazodone is used to facilitate sleep, as is amitriptyline, although the latter is less commonly used for this purpose. Venlafaxine can be used to reduce hot flashes that are a consequence of hormonal treatment for breast cancer. Lorazepam and some antipsychotics are frequently used as second- or third-line medications for nausea management in patients undergoing chemotherapy. Amphetamines are sometimes used in a time-limited fashion to address the severe fatigue that can accompany cancer treatment, but the SSRIs are more commonly used to help with fatigue, especially when fatigue is secondary to anxiety or depression.

4.1.4   Future Directions

Cannabis

Cannabis is a general term to describe compounds containing cannabinoids in various ratios. The most common cannabinoids are delta-9-tetrahydrocannabinol (THC) and cannabidiol (CBD), though more than 100 compounds have been isolated. At the federal level, cannabis/marijuana is listed on Schedule 1 of the Controlled Substances Act, making it illegal to possess. Schedule 1 drugs have no current accepted medical use. Despite federal regulations, some states have legalized cannabis for medicinal and recreational use.

> Cannabis is legal for medicinal and recreational use by some states but remains illegal at the federal level Because of a lack of robust, peer-reviewed evidence, the use of cannabinoids remains controversial

As cannabis becomes increasingly available, research has focused on its potential as a therapeutic agent. High-quality positive studies for the use of various cannabinoids in the treatment of depression and anxiety are generally lacking. This is attributable to existing regulations that have severely limited research in this emerging area, and the lack of uniformity in the cannabinoids being studied. At present, cannabis products are not considered to be an effective long-term treatment for depression or anxiety. However, this may change as cannabinoids become increasingly accessible and more studies emerge on the potential therapeutic benefits of these compounds. Although these drugs may provide temporary relief of these symptoms, there is also risk for a rebound or worsening depression or anxiety.

Cannabinoids have been utilized as monotherapy or in combination with other medications, with varying degrees of effectiveness, for the treatment of multiple symptoms associated with cancer (Romero-Sandoval et al., 2018;

Whiting et al., 2015). Additionally, cannabinoids have been useful in reducing the need for higher doses of opioids and in helping patients transition off opioid therapy (Nielsen et al., 2017). Medical cannabis is often managed by palliative care and medical oncology providers. Cannabis also has been associated with modest improvements in appetite for patients experiencing anorexia. In combination with other medications, cannabis can be a useful augmentation strategy in patients with refractory nausea and vomiting. However, excessive cannabis use may lead to a worsening of nausea and vomiting. Additionally, there is some evidence for the short-term use of cannabis products for insomnia. However, it is important to rule out other potential causes of insomnia before the initiation of cannabis as insomnia may be attributable to pain, and an underlying psychiatric disorder, or medication side effect.

More research is needed to determine the effectiveness of cannabis for pain, nausea, anorexia, and insomnia

Psilocybin

Psilocybin is a psychoactive substance derived from a variety of mushroom species. Historically, it was used by indigenous people of Central and South America as a part of their spiritual practices. Psilocybin is considered a psychedelic drug. Like cannabis, it is listed on Schedule 1 of the Controlled Substances Act. As of this writing, psilocybin has not been legalized in any state for recreational use. The mechanism of action for the psychedelic experience occurs via the serotonergic pathways of the central nervous system. Recently, psilocybin was investigated as an experimental drug for patients with cancer as an adjunctive treatment, along with psychotherapy, for mood, anxiety, and adjustment disorders (Reiff et al., 2020). In clinical trials, benefits were observed as soon as 1 month after the initial dose and sustained up to 6 months (the end of the monitoring period). In terminal cancer, psilocybin-assisted psychotherapy also led to reductions in reported depressive and anxiety symptoms up to 6 months (Reiff et al., 2020). In each of these studies, the clinical benefits were seen after a single dose. The use of psilocybin remains isolated to clinical trials and is not yet approved or readily available for clinical use.

MDMA

Methylenedioxymethamphetamine (MDMA) is the active substance of the drug of abuse commonly known as ecstasy. Like psilocybin, MDMA is a Schedule 1 drug and has not been legalized in any state for recreational use. Its mechanism of action is complex. Some of the psychoactive properties are mediated through the serotonin pathways of the central nervous system, like that of psilocybin. Additionally, some of its psychoactive properties resemble those of other stimulants such as amphetamines, including methamphetamine, which influence activity in the dopamine and norepinephrine pathways. MDMA has shown some benefit in medication-assisted therapy in patients with PTSD, and clinical trials are currently underway to explore its use with other anxiety disorders and anxiety associated with a terminal illness (Reiff et al., 2020). MDMA has yet to be utilized as an investigational drug for patients with cancer. Given the early clinical benefits seen with psilocybin in this patient population – and the clinical benefits observed in patients who have experienced trauma – MDMA will likely have clinical applicability in this patient population in the future.

Collaborative Care

Collaborative care models are evidence-based, team-based approaches to mental-health treatment which increase access to treatment and improve psychiatric symptoms for patients in oncology settings (Fann et al., 2012; Li et al., 2017; Sharpe et al., 2014). Collaborative care is designed to provide rapid access to cost-effective assessment and treatment. These models can also be extended to serious mental illness and cancer (Irwin et al., 2019). Collaborative care psychiatry is a patient-centered, integrated medical-behavioral model for delivering psychiatric care to patients in medical environments, where access to psychiatric care is often quite limited.

Collaborative care is an efficient and effective model for the delivery of mental-health treatment

Collaborative care relies on a team-based approach, incorporating the primary medical team, the psychiatrist, and the behavioral health manager (BHM). The BHM is often a licensed clinical social worker or psychiatric registered nurse who has prior training in evidence-based brief-psychotherapeutic interventions. In this model of care, the primary medical team is responsible for screening and identifying patients with acute distress and psychiatric symptoms. The patient is assessed by the BHM, and the case is discussed with the consulting psychiatrist to formulate a treatment plan. The primary team then partners with the patient, the BHM, and the psychiatrist to implement recommendations for psychiatric treatment, including writing the prescriptions for psychiatric medications. In oncology, the medical oncologist occupies the role of the primary medical provider, with the psychiatrist as a consultant. The responsibilities of the BHM include the initial psychiatric evaluation, weekly case consultation with the psychiatrist, and communication with the primary medical team. The BHM follows up with the patient at regular intervals and measures progress using the patient interview as well as evidence-based standardized assessment tools specific to the patient's diagnosis. The BHM may provide brief psychotherapeutic interventions as needed. Common brief psychotherapeutic interventions include motivational interviewing, behavioral activation, or brief CBT for pain or insomnia. If the patient's symptoms are in remission, the patient and BHM create a relapse-prevention plan, and the patient is transitioned into routine care. The psychiatric consultant is responsible for participating in weekly case consultation, providing pharmacologic and psychotherapeutic treatment recommendations, and for direct consultation with the primary medical team as needed. If a patient does not improve with this intervention, then the patient is referred into the traditional direct-care model of psychiatric treatment and is evaluated and followed up by a psychiatrist.

The collaborative care team includes the patient, the oncologist, the behavioral health manager, and the psychiatrist

Patients are often excluded from collaborative care if they have more severe psychiatric needs such as bipolar disorder, primary psychotic disorders (schizophrenia or schizoaffective disorder), severe SUDs, treatment-resistant depression or anxiety, or a long-standing history of recurrent or refractory mental illness. However, in locations where psychiatric resources are scarce, collaborative care can guide treatment in these cases.

Collaborative care has been implemented in many medical environments, with the greatest success seen in the management of major depression. In oncology, the oncologist occupies the role of the primary medical provider. Uncontrolled psychiatric symptoms in patients with cancer can lead to lower adherence to cancer treatment, worse health and QoL outcomes, and increased utilization of medical services (Kisely et al., 2013; Paredes et al., 2021). Collaborative care has been shown to improve each of these outcomes while reducing the wait time for access to mental-health treatment.

4.2   Effectiveness of Treatments

4.2.1   Psychosocial Interventions

A recent review of online interventions for individuals who had completed treatment for cancer demonstrated that CBT was the most common intervention utilized (Willems et al., 2020). CBT interventions were beneficial in terms of decreased fear of cancer recurrence, decreased insomnia, improved sleep quality, and decreased memory difficulties. Online interventions were determined to be accessible and acceptable to cancer survivors.

In a meta-analysis of mindfulness interventions with cancer patients, evidence was found for improvements in QoL, anxiety, depression, and some physical symptoms (fatigue, sleep) (Haller at al., 2017). In another review of studies with cancer patients, use of acceptance and commitment therapy was found to be associated with better mood and QoL (González-Fernández & Fernández-Rodríguez, 2019). Finally, in a review of interventions with colorectal cancer patients, emotional expression, progressive muscle relaxation training, and interventions focused on self-efficacy demonstrated a significant positive impact on mental health (Mosher et al., 2017).

A recent review of psychosocial interventions for patients with advanced cancer included these interventions: CBT, meaning-centered therapy, dignity therapy, supportive counseling, psychoeducation, and integrative therapies (e.g., music, writing) (Teo et al., 2019). CBT was determined to benefit QoL, relevant symptoms (pain, fatigue, shortness of breath), and self-efficacy. Meaning-centered therapies were also found to be effective, with benefits in QoL and spiritual well-being. Dignity therapy was found to be effective in terms of decreased distress.

4.2.2   Psychotropic Medications

With all psychiatric medications, the goal of treatment is full remission of symptoms. Not all patients, however, achieve full remission, therefore ongoing assessment and management are required.

Effectiveness of Antidepressants for Depression
In the general population, antidepressants significantly improve depressive symptoms of major depressive disorder compared to placebo as early as 4 weeks after treatment initiation (Cipriani et al., 2011). Treatment response rates to a single antidepressant (measured as a 50% reduction in depressive symptoms on validated scales) are estimated to be as high as 60% by 12 weeks compared to a 41% response rate for placebo (Cipriani et al.). When a patient has a clinical response to an antidepressant, they demonstrate a reduction in

Antidepressants are effective in reducing overall severity of depression symptoms

the severity of symptoms and experience some relief. However, the goal of treatment remains remission: Patients who achieve remission are less likely to have future episodes of depression than those with persistent symptoms. Therefore, it is important to continue treatment beyond a clinical response and strive for full remission. Rates of remission (measured by achieving a subthreshold score on validated scales) after one or more successive trials of antidepressants are estimated to be as high as 67% (Rush et al., 2006). Many patients require more than one trial of medication to achieve remission, and some patients require a combination of medications to achieve remission. One challenge regarding the use of psychiatric medications for psychiatric illness is that many patients never get beyond the first trial of medication, leading to lower rates of remission than might have been achieved with ongoing participation in treatment. Barriers to longitudinal participation in treatment include problems with regular or frequent access to psychiatric providers, intolerable side effects of medications, improvement in symptoms leading to self-discontinuation of treatment, or treatment failure leading to reduced confidence in the potential benefit of alternative medications. Approximately one-third of patients have a treatment response but will not achieve full remission. The rates of recurrence for major depressive episodes increase with each successive episode. For example, after the first episode, there is a 50% chance of recurrence over the patient's lifetime if they reach remission and discontinue their medication. This rate increases to 70% if the patient has had two episodes and 90% if the patient has had three or more episodes. As mentioned in Chapter 3, few clinical trials have investigated the effectiveness of antidepressants in patients with cancer, and more research is needed in this population. In general, no single antidepressant is considered superior to any other medication. The choice of antidepressant is made based on clinical judgment when considering target symptoms, avoiding drug interactions with anticancer medications, and paying close attention to effectiveness and tolerability.

Treatment for depression can be challenging and may require multiple attempts with one or more medications

Evidence for antidepressants in cancer patients is limited, and medication choice is based on clinical judgment

Effectiveness of Antidepressants in GAD

Antidepressants are an effective treatment for GAD (Slee et al., 2019). Treatment response rates (measured as a 50% reduction in anxiety symptoms on validated scales) to a single antidepressant can be as high as 73%, compared to placebo response rates which can be as high as 45% (Gale et al., 2011). Rates of remission (measured by achieving a subthreshold score on validated scales) after a single trial of an antidepressant may be as high as 36% compared to placebo, for which the response may be as high as 19% (Gale et al., 2011). Often antidepressants are used in combination with benzodiazepines or antihistamines to control symptoms of anxiety. As with major depression, few clinical trials have investigated the use of antidepressants for anxiety disorder in patients with cancer.

Antidepressants are effective in reducing symptoms of anxiety

Antidepressants are often prescribed in combination with other medications to further reduce symptoms of anxiety

Effectiveness of Antidepressants in Panic Disorder

Antidepressants are an effective treatment for panic disorder (Bighelli et al., 2018). Treatment response rates (measured as a 50% reduction in depressive symptoms on validated scales) to a single antidepressant can be as high as 60% compared to placebo response rates as high as 45% (Bighelli et al.). Rates of remission (measured by achieving a subthreshold score on validated scales) after a single trial of an antidepressant can be as high as 49% compared to placebo which may be as high as 40% (Bighelli et al.).

Effectiveness of Antidepressants in PTSD

Antidepressants are an effective treatment for PTSD (Watts et al., 2013). Treatment response rates (measured as a 50% reduction in depressive symptoms on validated scales) to a single antidepressant can be as high as 59% compared to placebo response rates as high as 38% (Tucker et al., 2001). Rates of remission (measured by achieving a subthreshold score on validated scales) after a single trial of an antidepressant may be as high as 30% compared to placebo, which may be as high as 15% (Davidson, 2004). In general, no single antidepressant is considered superior to any other medication.

4.3   Challenges in Delivering Treatment

4.3.1   Access Concerns for Treatment

Patients face many barriers to accessing mental-health treatment, and patients with cancer are no exception. Because of the nature of their complex medical problems, these patients may have significant financial challenges or "financial toxicity." Financial toxicity is associated with poor QoL, reduced adherence to treatment, and worse treatment outcomes (Alcaraz et al., 2020). Often patients are unable to maintain full employment during their cancer treatment, which makes it more difficult for them to pay for housing, food, and medications. Further, limitations in employment may impede a patient's ability to maintain health insurance. In the US, even with health insurance coverage, individuals may have only limited benefits for mental-health treatment. At times, their insurance may require large copayments for such treatments or limit which providers are covered (psychiatrist, psychologist, licensed clinical social worker). Additionally, coverage for mental-health treatment may only be approved for specific locations where a patient can receive care. Including social workers, case managers, or navigators on the treatment team can help in addressing some of the financial barriers patients face while receiving cancer treatments.

Patients with cancer may encounter problems with access to mental-health treatment

Some patients will have difficulty traveling to and from appointments because of multiple barriers. Some patients may have to travel great distances to receive their cancer treatment; the time involved in transportation limits their ability to participate in mental-health treatment because they may feel as though they only have time for cancer treatment appointments. Additionally, in less populous areas, access to mental-health treatment is historically challenging because of limited providers and providers with already closed caseloads being unable to accommodate new patients. Not all patients have access to personal vehicles to travel to and from appointments and thus may have to rely on others to provide transportation. In large urban centers, public transportation may be an option, but is not always feasible because of the amount of time it takes to utilize this resource. Other barriers to public transportation may

Telemedicine is emerging as an effective way to increase access to mental-health treatment

include the patient's physical limitations and concerns related to exposure to pathogens while in an immunocompromised state. In rural and suburban areas, public transportation may be quite limited, if it is available at all. Patients likely feel the need to prioritize opportunities for transportation assistance for their oncology-related appointments and may not be able to obtain additional transportation for mental-health appointments. The emergence of telemedicine as a treatment modality for mental health can help overcome some of the barriers posed by lack of access to timely and adequate transportation.

4.3.2   Presence of Family/Caretakers

As alluded to in the above section, patients must often rely on family members, friends, and caretakers for financial, transportation, and emotional support during their cancer treatment. It is common for these individuals to accompany patients to their appointments. At times, patients request that support persons be included in mental-health treatment similar to their involvement in other areas of their cancer treatment. This involvement provides a unique opportunity to learn more about patients and their circumstances. It also allows another historian to report symptoms, setbacks, and progress. It is important to work effectively with both parties to improve outcomes. Some caretakers are accustomed to assuming the role of the primary reporter as well as decision-maker. This adaptive role may sometimes be more beneficial in the oncology setting than it is in the mental-health setting. Caretakers may inadvertently speak for patients or make assumptions about patient symptoms that are not always accurate, which can lead to inaccurate diagnoses, incomplete treatment plans, and delays in patient progress. In these situations, it may be useful to separate the patient from the caretaker for an individualized assessment. When the assessment is complete, the clinician can then invite the caretaker to join for the remainder of the appointment. It is important to engage the patient in taking an active role in their treatment as opposed to relying solely on the caretaker, which serves to empower the patient, promote self-efficacy for medical management, and minimize the burden on supportive parties. Additionally, patients should be allowed to identify specific information as confidential that will not be shared with the caretaker. Sometimes, the nature of this confidentiality is obvious; other times it is worthwhile to engage the patient in a discussion regarding their desire to withhold certain information from the caretaker, especially when the clinician believes the sharing of such information could benefit the patient and the caretaker.

Caretakers are at high risk for distress and burnout

It is common for caretakers to experience elevated levels of stress because of a multitude of factors including financial concerns, increasing demands for patient care because of increased patient disability, modifications to family roles and responsibilities, difficulty coping with the patient's diagnosis and prognosis, and end-of-life concerns. At times, conflicts may arise between the patient and their caretakers because of the nature of this relationship. Patients may feel guilty or feel they are becoming a burden to those helping them. This can be a symptom of, or contribute to, adjustment disorders, depression, and anxiety disorders. Caretakers face the risk of burnout because of increasing demands placed on them by the patient's clinical situation and the length of time they may be needed to provide care. Also, some caretakers may feel uncomfortable with medical settings or medical care, increasing the opportunity for guilty feelings if they try to set limits on caregiving duties.

4.3.3   High Burden of Disease

For some patients, early detection of cancer leads to definitive treatment without long-lasting needs for ongoing surveillance and treatment. However, many patients are diagnosed at later stages of their disease or experience recurrence, leading to the concept of cancer as a chronic disease that worsens over time and requires ongoing treatment to prolong survival. These patients will face an increasing burden of disease, with growing physical limitations that may make it more difficult to attend regular visits, limit endurance for mental health treatment sessions, or impair ability to effectively communicate during mental health sessions. In these instances, it is often helpful to partner with palliative care providers who are experts at managing symptoms and high levels of disease burden. The goal is to reduce physical, emotional, and psychological suffering. Greater physical comfort may also prolong the patient's ability to engage in mental-health treatment and improve their overall QoL.

4.3.4   The Therapist's Personal Experience With Cancer

Cancer touches the lives of all people, and mental-health providers are no exception. Providers may have direct experience as cancer patients or as caretakers, which can increase their ability to relate to their patients. Alternatively, this experience may increase their risk for re-exposure to their own trauma as they engage with this patient population. Similarly, providers may themselves be current or past caretakers for family members or friends who have had cancer. Providing care to this patient population may stir negative emotions and memories in the mental-health provider and may color their treatment of patients – both positively and negatively. As is the case when treating the general population, mental-health providers should be mindful of their own biases, emotions, memories, and experiences, and understand how these factors may impact patient care. If the mental-health provider is having a particularly strong emotional reaction to a patient, they should explore why this is the case. Providers can and should consider seeking out regular supervision to explore these reactions and learn skills to manage them better to improve patient care.

Providers must consider their own experiences with cancer and understand how these may impact their ability to care for patients

4.3.5   Burnout/Compassion Fatigue

There is a growing awareness of the prevalence of burnout and compassion fatigue in healthcare professionals. Psycho-oncology providers may experience this as well. In a survey of 417 psychosocial oncology clinicians from 10 international and national professional societies, burnout was determined to be a problem in 45% of psychologists, 32% of social workers, 7% of psychiatrists, 4% of counselors, and 12% of allied health professionals (Rasmussen et al., 2016). Across the full cohort, 20% reported high emotional exhaustion, and 7% reported high depersonalization on the Maslach Burnout Inventory. The American Psychological Association published an article on self-care and recommended the following strategies for coping with the strains of difficult clinical work: (1) observing your own stress levels and practicing basic self-care (sufficient sleep, healthy diet, regular exercise); (2) proactively addressing stress; (3) setting boundaries around your work to preserve some work-life balance; (4) seeking and utilizing social supports; and (5) practicing self-compassion (Abramson, 2021).

4.3.6   End-of-Life Care

Dying patients often require special attention for their physical, emotional, psychological, and spiritual needs. Medical care at the end of life can involve increasing reliance on palliative care (holistic care focused on relieving symptoms and promoting QoL) or referral to hospice care (holistic care delivered without curative intent for those patients with a life expectancy of fewer than 6 months). Mental-health interventions, both psychotherapeutic and psychopharmacological, can be delivered as a component of palliative care and/or hospice care, or as an adjunct to either. Patients have asserted that a good death is associated with dying quickly, with minimal suffering, without dependence on others, but with interpersonal relations preserved (Kastbom et al., 2017). Additional concerns relating to psychological and spiritual functioning can include the desire for a feeling of closure, reflection on personal values, optimization of relationships, clarifying legacy, and affirming religious beliefs. Supportive and existential interventions can be useful in helping patients and their support persons process anticipatory grief and bereavement.

4.4   Multicultural Issues

4.4.1   Diversity Issues

Historically, access to appropriate screening, early detection, and treatment of cancer has been unequal across racial groups. Racial and ethnic differences in rates of screening and early detection of breast and colorectal cancers are well documented (Berland et al., 2019). This has led to a greater prevalence of advanced disease and higher rates of morbidity and mortality in underrepresented populations. The same groups have also had unequal access to mental-health treatment and have faced biases when accessing treatment. Combining these two major concerns, patients from underrepresented groups face significant challenges when confronted with the diagnosis of cancer and are at risk for higher rates of distress and mental-health problems. Oncology programs and associated mental-health providers must be mindful of these historic inequities and take proactive efforts to mitigate these.

4.4.2   Religious Beliefs and Decision-Making About Treatment

For many patients, the presence or absence of religious and spiritual beliefs impacts decision-making regarding treatment. The patient's belief structure may determine which treatments are acceptable, how the patient approaches end-of-life, and which coping strategies the patient may rely on at each transition point in the cancer continuum. It is important to screen for the presence or absence of religious or spiritual beliefs during the initial encounters to obtain a greater understanding of the patient. Providers may ask questions such as, "Do you consider yourself a religious or spiritual person?", "What role do your religious or spiritual beliefs play in your life?", "How do your religious or spiritual beliefs interact with your current situation?" Mental-health providers can leverage the skills of religious leaders or chaplains to further support their patients. These individuals may also help guide the mental-health provider's and the patient's understanding of end-of-life and existential concerns and ease suffering around these issues.

5

Case Vignettes

5.1   Case Vignette 1: Ms. R.

Ms. R. is a 62-year-old, single, African American female with a history of breast cancer, for which she was treated with double mastectomy with reconstruction and chemotherapy approximately 3 years before presenting for psychotherapy. She was referred to psychosocial oncology for the management of pain and mood disturbance. At the time of her initial evaluation, she had not returned to work since receiving her initial cancer diagnosis and was receiving social security disability payments. Ms. R.'s chief complaint was, "I just want to get rid of the pain. And I want to be my pre-cancer self."

Ms. R. reported the onset of symptoms of depression around the time she started chemotherapy, significantly worsening in the 2–3 months before presenting for evaluation after a wrist injury. She described experiencing persistent low mood, lack of pleasure from previously enjoyable activities, reduced motivation, limited energy and fatigue, feelings of hopelessness about the future, thoughts of worthlessness because of her inability to return to work, frequent crying, insomnia, emotional eating, and social isolation. She reported sleeping about 3 hours per night and identified pain at her chest wall and mastectomy incision sites as the cause of her frequent awakenings. Ms. R. admitted that she had stopped sleeping in her bedroom, preferring to sleep on the couch. She explained that at some point since undergoing her diagnostic workup, she had started to find her bedroom claustrophobic. She described having passive thoughts of suicide, such as, "I wish I could go to sleep and not wake up," but she denied ever having a suicidal plan and noted she would not act on her thoughts because of her concerns for her daughter and her religious beliefs.

Ms. R. also described feeling increasingly anxious over the last 3 years, initially with uncontrollable worry about her cancer, and later with more pervasive and generalized anxiety. She reported feeling persistently nervous, with uncontrollable, excessive worry about the future. She felt irritable, had poor concentration, and experienced physical symptoms of anxiety such as heart racing, stomach upset, and, on a few occasions, hyperventilation. Ms. R. provided a detailed account of her anxiety triggers, which included being around other people, leaving her home, sleeping in her bedroom, having acute pain flares, and seeing or touching her breasts. She was dissatisfied with the results of her reconstructive surgery and described taking several measures to avoid looking at her breasts, including covering the mirrors in her home and only looking up while bathing. She frequently remarked, "I look like a monster now," and worried that when she is in public, people stare at her to try to discern whether or not her breasts are "real." She also described withdrawing from her social network because of a few experiences in which she felt others were insensitive about her experiences.

Ms. R. spent most of her day taking medication, shopping online, watching television, and snacking. She only left home for medical appointments, relying on her daughter to bring food, medications, and other household necessities. Before her cancer diagnosis, Ms. R. worked as an administrative assistant and took pride in her work. She also had a robust social network and described "running a tight ship" at home. She lived alone in a single-family home in a neighborhood with high rates of gun violence – another significant source of stress for her. She was never married, although she was in a long-term intimate relationship that ended when she informed her significant other of her cancer diagnosis. She had one daughter (30 years old). Ms. R. was an only child, and her parents were deceased. At the time of her initial evaluation, she identified her daughter as a strong source of support but felt guilty about the burden she was placing on her. Nonetheless, she avoided reaching out to her friends and church community, despite their many efforts to connect with her. She believed she would never be able to return to work or achieve her pre-cancer level of functioning because of her pain, depression, and anxiety. Ms. R. was unable to generate any coping strategies that she found useful for managing her symptoms, though she was drinking up to three beers per day to help her relax.

Ms. R. denied having any psychiatric history before her cancer diagnosis and treatments. She briefly met with a psychiatrist for medication management of her mood symptoms right after completing treatment, but she was nonadherent with her medications and appointments. She did not believe the medications were helpful and "wasn't ready" to engage in mental-health treatment at that time.

Ms. R. was pleasant during the evaluation, though she was somewhat withdrawn and guarded, and she struggled to maintain eye contact. She was appropriately dressed and groomed. Her speech was soft and slow. Her mood was depressed with flat affect congruent with her reported symptoms. She completed several scales evaluating mood, coping, cognitive functioning, and pain (see Table 10).

Conceptualization and Considerations for Treatment Planning

- Ms. R. has been minimally engaged in mental-health treatment, despite her pain and mood symptoms persisting for over 3 years.
- The impact of Ms. R.'s mood symptoms and pain on her functioning and cancer survivorship experience is significant.
- Ms. R. utilizes avoidant coping strategies and exhibits a tendency toward helplessness, which serve to maintain her mood and anxiety symptoms and reinforce her unhelpful beliefs about pain.
- Ms. R.'s sociocultural context, such as living in a high-violence neighborhood, appears to contribute to her overall distress.

Table 10
Assessment Tools Used to Assess Ms. R

Scale administered	Score	Diagnostic/implication
BDI-II	42/63	Severe depression
BAI	28/63	Moderately severe anxiety
Columbia Suicide Severity Rating Scale	N/A	Passive SI in past
Pain Catastrophizing Scale	52/52	Significant rumination, magnification, helplessness
Insomnia Severity Index	22/28	Clinical insomnia (severe)
Penn State Worry Questionnaire	48/80	Moderate worry
Brief COPE	Multiple scales	Frequent use of substance use, behavioral disengagement, venting, religion, and self-blame; infrequent use of active coping, planning, and positive reframing
Mini Mental Status Exam (MMSE)	26/30	No cognitive impairment; appropriate attention, concentration, registration, and recall
West Haven-Yale Multidimensional Pain Inventory	Multiple scales	High interference in activity, low support, high affective distress, predominant use of negative responses

Diagnostic Impressions

- Major Depressive Disorder, Single Episode, Severe
- Generalized Anxiety Disorder
- Agoraphobia
- Cancer-related pain

Treatment Plan

Ms. R. identified the following goals for treatment:
- Increase activity level
- Increase social interaction
- Learn how to manage pain
- Explore issues related to cancer survivorship and self-esteem

She agreed to the following treatment plan:
- Treatment with her psychiatrist to revisit recommendations for starting an antidepressant.

- Psychoeducation on the relationship between cancer diagnosis, treatment, and survivorship and psychological distress, and on the relationship between pain and mood.
- Behavioral activation for depression, incorporating behavioral strategies for pain management, such as pacing scheduled activities.
- Relaxation strategies for acute symptoms of anxiety.
- Cognitive behavioral therapy for depression, anxiety, and chronic pain. Learning and implementing cognitive strategies to address pain appraisals/pain catastrophizing and restructuring distorted beliefs about herself and her body, other people, and the world.
- Exposure therapy using a hierarchy to address salient anxiety triggers (sleeping in the bedroom, leaving the house, being around other people).

Response to Treatment

Ms. R. completed 22 sessions of psychotherapy. She re-established care with her psychiatrist and started an antidepressant with a good symptom response. She found that her motivation and energy had improved, which allowed her to engage more meaningfully with interventions in psychotherapy. The first several sessions focused on behavioral activation for depression and learning relaxation and grounding techniques for anxiety. She was able to apply several of these skills to pain management, and while she continued to struggle with pain, she felt more empowered to apply nonpharmacological strategies to improve functioning. Ms. R. was initially hesitant to move forward with exposure-based interventions, but eventually elicited her daughter's support to encourage her and hold her accountable. She achieved her goals of sleeping in her bedroom, looking at her breasts, and attending a handful of small social events.

5.2   Case Vignette 2: Mr. J.

Mr. J. is a 44-year-old married, Caucasian male who was diagnosed 6 months ago with oropharyngeal squamous cell carcinoma after presenting to his primary-care physician with a sore throat that failed to go away. Further workup with an oncologist revealed the cancer was locally advanced, and the biopsy indicated the cancer was HPV-positive. He underwent surgery and was referred to psychosocial oncology for "family conflict" shortly after initiating adjuvant chemotherapy and radiation.

During his first session, Mr. J. stated he did not see why he needed to meet with a psychologist and was only attending at the urging of his wife. He endorsed feeling "angry" about his situation. He remarked several times that he saw providers who had failed to further investigate his sore throat and felt strongly that if he had been "taken seriously," his cancer would have been identified sooner. Mr. J. was particularly upset about his gastric feeding tube, which he had received at the time of his cancer resection to ensure adequate nutritional intake. He reported arguing with his wife several times per day about completing his tube feeds, although he admitted he was struggling to get enough nutrition orally and was losing weight. He described spending most of the day sitting in his chair in front of the TV, and he had been turning down offers for visits from friends. He worried they would pity him when they saw his surgery scars and weight loss and heard about the burdens of chemotherapy and radiation. He became remorseful when discussing his recent tendency to lash out at his children and stated he had had little patience for anything since his surgery. Mr. J. reported feeling embarrassed by the fact that his cancer was HPV-positive. He described ruminating over partners before his wife, convinced he had been sexually irresponsible in some way. Mr. J. stated at times that he feels so guilty he can barely look his wife in the eye. He stated, "I hate that she needs to take care of me. It's mortifying. I am supposed to be the man of the household. And I could have made her sick on top of everything else."

Mr. J. was working as a foreman for a construction firm before he learned of his diagnosis. He left work on short-term disability but resisted applying for Family Medical Leave Act (FMLA) benefits as he hoped to return to work as soon as possible. He described loving his work and relished being a person who could fix anything with his own hands. He lived in a small house with his wife of 15 years, their two children (a 14-year-old boy and a 9-year-old girl), and a dog. His father was deceased, while his mother, brother, and sister all lived nearby. Mr. J. was close with them and expressed appreciation for their support of his wife during this difficult time.

Mr. J. reported one possible depressive episode when he was in his twenties, shortly after his father had died of pancreatic cancer. He did not receive any treatment at the time. He otherwise denied any psychiatric history. He reported smoking about half a pack of cigarettes per day since he was 18 but had been using a nicotine patch since his surgery and reported frequent cravings to smoke. He described drinking approximately two beers after work most days and up to six beers per day on the weekend. He denied any history of blackouts, withdrawal symptoms, driving violations, or other problems as a result of his alcohol use, though he stated his wife had been encouraging him to cut back for years. He admitted to having "a few beers" since his surgery. He denied any history of drug use.

Mr. J. was initially irritable and guarded during the evaluation. Nonetheless, he verbalized willingness to schedule a follow-up visit.

Conceptualization and Considerations for Treatment Planning

- Mr. J. is ambivalent about participating in treatment, though he does have insight into the impact of his cancer diagnosis and treatments on his mood, behavior, and relationships.
- Mr. J. is struggling with significant identity and role changes that contribute to his feelings of anger and depressed presentation.
- Mr. J. can clearly articulate his values across multiple domains, but he repeatedly moves away from his values in an attempt to avoid painful thoughts and emotions.
- Mr. J.'s tobacco and alcohol use requires ongoing monitoring and intervention.

Diagnostic Impressions

- Adjustment disorder with depressed mood
- Tobacco use disorder, in early remission
- R/O alcohol use disorder, mild

Treatment Plan

Over the next few sessions, Mr. J. identified the following goals for treatment:
- Increase level of physical activity, including identifying ways to contribute around the house.
- Implement health behavior changes, such as limiting the use of alcohol, remaining abstinent from tobacco use, and improving diet/nutrition.
- Improve communication with his wife, children, and other social supports.
- Modify unhelpful thoughts of self-blame regarding his cancer.

Response to Treatment

Mr. J. continued to be ambivalent about treatment intermittently and ultimately terminated psychotherapy before meaningfully addressing his unhelpful cognitions or consistently reducing his tobacco use. However, he did demonstrate improvements in behavioral activation, specifically by establishing and maintaining a daily schedule that included mild physical activity and assisting with household chores. He reported improvement in motivation and energy because of these behavior changes. Mr. J. also engaged with interventions for promoting assertive communication, which helped him to better communicate emotional needs to his family and to reduce the frequency of angry outbursts.

6

Further Reading

Breitbart, W. (2014). *Psychosocial palliative care.* Oxford University Press. https://doi.org/10.1093/med/9780199917402.001.0001
This book addresses psychosocial care of patients with advanced illness. It covers psychotherapeutic and psychopharmacologic interventions.

Holland, J. C. (Ed.). (2010). *Psycho-oncology.* Oxford University Press. https://doi.org/10.1093/med/9780195367430.001.0001
This fundamental guide is written by experts in the field of psycho-oncology. It is a comprehensive in-depth review of all aspects of psycho-oncology.

Holland, J. C., & Lewis, S. (2000). *The human side of cancer: Living with hope, coping with uncertainty.* HarperCollins.
This book addresses the patient perspective on cancer and its treatment. It provides useful grounding in the patient experience.

Kabat-Zinn, J. (2013). *Full catastrophe living: Using the wisdom of your body and mind to face stress, pain, and illness.* Bantam.
This book is based on Kabat-Zinn's mindfulness-based stress reduction model. It presents mind–body approaches to promote well-being and health.

Riba, M. B., Donovan, K. A., Andersen, B., Braun, I., Breitbart, W. S., Brewer, B. W., Buchmann, L. O., Clark, M. M., Collins, M., Corbett, C., Fleishman, S., Garcia, S., Greenberg, D. B., Handzo, G. F., Hoofring, L., Huang, C., Lally, R., Martin, S., McGuffey, L., … Darlow, S. D. (2019). Distress management, version 3.2019, NCCN clinical practice guidelines in oncology. *Journal of the National Comprehensive Cancer Network, 17*(10), 1229–1249. https://doi.org/10.6004/jnccn.2019.0048
This summary provides an overview of distress management and the evidence-based treatment pathways detailed in the NCCN Distress Management Guidelines.

7

References

Abramson, A. (2021). The ethical imperative of self-care. *Monitor on Psychology, 52*(3), 46–53.

Ader, R., & Cohen, N. (1975). Behaviorally conditioned immunosuppression. *Psychosomatic Medicine, 37*(4), 333–340. https://doi.org/10.1097/00006842-197507000-00007

Adler, N. E., Page, A., & Institute of Medicine (US) Committee on Psychosocial Services to Cancer Patients/Families in a Community Setting (Eds.). (2008). *Cancer care for the whole patient: Meeting psychosocial health needs.* National Academies Press (US).

Akechi, T., Okuyama, T., Onishi, J., Morita, T., & Furukawa, T. A. (2008). Psychotherapy for depression among incurable cancer patients. *The Cochrane database of systematic reviews, 2008*(2), CD005537. https://doi.org/10.1002/14651858.CD005537.pub2

Alcaraz, K. I., Wiedt, T. L., Daniels, E. C., Yabroff, K. R., Guerra, C. E., & Wender, R. C. (2020). Understanding and addressing social determinants to advance cancer health equity in the United States: A blueprint for practice, research, and policy. *CA: A Cancer Journal for Clinicians, 70*(1), 31–46. https://doi.org/10.3322/caac.21586

American Cancer Society (ACS). (2019). *Cancer facts and figures 2019.* Author.

American Psychiatric Association (APA). (2013). *Diagnostic and statistical manual of mental disorders* (5th ed.). Author.

Antoni, M. H., Lechner, S., Diaz, A., Vargas, S., Holley, H., Phillips, K., McGregor, B., Carver, C. S., & Blomberg, B. (2009). Cognitive behavioral stress management effects on psychosocial and physiological adaptation in women undergoing treatment for breast cancer. *Brain, Behavior, & Immunity, 23*(5), 580–591. https://doi.org/10.1016/j.bbi.2008.09.005

Annas, G. J. (2017). *Health law* (Encyclopedia Britannica). https://www.britannica.com/science/health-law

Applebaum, A. J., & Breitbart, W. (2013). Care for the cancer caregiver: A systematic review. *Palliative & Supportive Care, 11*(3), 231–252. https://doi.org/10.1017/S1478951512000594

Asher, A., & Myers, J. S. (2015). The effect of cancer treatment on cognitive function. *Clinical Advances in Hematology & Oncology, 13*(7), 441–450.

Atkins, G. T., Kim, T., & Munson, J. (2017). Residence in rural areas of the United States and lung cancer mortality: Disease incidence, treatment disparities, and stage-specific survival. *Annals of the American Thoracic Society, 14*(3), 403–411. https://doi.org/10.1513/AnnalsATS.201606-4690

Baik, O. M., & Adams, K. B. (2011). Improving the well-being of couples facing cancer: A review of couples-based psychosocial interventions. *Journal of Marital and Family Therapy, 37*(2), 250–266. https://doi.org/10.1111/j.1752-0606.2010.00217.x

Bauml, J. M., Troxel, A., Epperson, C. N., Cohen, R. B., Schmitz, K., Stricker, C., Shulman, L. N., Bradbury, A., Mao, J. J., & Langer, C. J. (2016). Scan-associated distress in lung cancer: Quantifying the impact of "scanxiety". *Lung Cancer, 100*, 110–113. https://doi.org/10.1016/j.lungcan.2016.08.002

Beck, A.T., Steer, R.A., Brown, G.K. (1996). *Manual for Beck Depression Inventory-II.* Psychological Corp.

Berland, L. L., Monticciolo, D. L., Flores, E. J., Malak, S. F., Yee, J., & Dyer, D. S. (2019). Relationships between healthcare disparities and coverage policies for breast, colon, and lung cancer screening. *Journal of the American College of Radiology, 16*(4 Pt B), 580–585. https://doi.org/10.1016/j.jacr.2018.12.025

Bighelli, I., Castellazzi, M., Cipriani, A., Girlanda, F., Guaiana, G., Koesters, M., Turrini, G., Furukawa, T. A., & Barbui, C. (2018). Antidepressants versus placebo for panic disorder in adults. *The Cochrane Database of Systematic Reviews, 4*(4), CD010676. https://doi.org/10.1002/14651858.CD010676.pub2

Bonanno G. A. (2004). Loss, trauma, and human resilience: have we underestimated the human capacity to thrive after extremely aversive events? *The American Psychologist, 59*(1), 20–28. https://doi.org/10.1037/0003-066X.59.1.20

Braun, D. P., Gupta, D., Grutsch, J. F., & Staren, E. D. (2011). Can changes in health related quality of life scores predict survival in stages III and IV colorectal cancer? *Health and Quality Of Life Outcomes, 9*, 62. https://doi.org/10.1186/1477-7525-9-62

Braun, D. P., Gupta, D., & Staren, E. D. (2013). Longitudinal health-related quality of life assessment implications for prognosis in stage IV pancreatic cancer. *Pancreas, 42*(2), 254–259. https://doi.org/10.1097/MPA.0b013e31825b9f56

Breitbart, W., Rosenfeld, B., Gibson, C., Pessin, H., Poppito, S., Nelson, C., Tomarken, A., Timm, A. K., Berg, A., Jacobson, C., Sorger, B., Abbey, J., & Olden, M. (2010). Meaning-centered group psychotherapy for patients with advanced cancer: A pilot randomized controlled trial. *Psycho-Oncology, 19*(1), 21–28. https://doi.org/10.1002/pon.1556

Breitbart, W., Pessin, H., Rosenfeld, B., Applebaum, A.J., Lichtenthal, W.G., Li, Y., Saracino, R.M., Marziliano, A.M., Masterson, M., Tobias, K., & Fenn, N. (2018). Individual meaning-centered psychotherapy for the treatment of psychological and existential distress: A randomized controlled trial in patients with advanced cancer. *Cancer, 124*(15), 3231–3239. https://doi.org/10.1002/cncr.31539

Brennan J. (2001). Adjustment to cancer – coping or personal transition? *Psycho-Oncology, 10*(1), 1–18. https://doi.org/10.1002/1099-1611(200101/02)10:1<1::aid-pon484>3.0.co;2-t

Bruera, E., Kuehn, N., Miller, M. J., Selmser, P., & Macmillan, K. (1991). The Edmonton Symptom Assessment System (ESAS): A simple method for the assessment of palliative care patients. *Journal of Palliative Care, 7*(2), 6–9. https://doi.org/10.1177/082585979100700202

Cancer.Net. (2019). *Long-term side effects of cancer treatment*. American Society of Clinical Oncology. https://www.cancer.net/survivorship/long-term-side-effects-cancer-treatment

Carlson, L., & Speca, M. (2011). *Mindfulness-based cancer recovery: A step-by-step MBSR approach to help you cope with treatment and reclaim your life*. New Harbinger Publications.

Cella, D. F., Tulsky, D. S., Gray, G., Sarafian, B., Linn, E., Bonomi, A., Silberman, M., Yellen, S. B., Winicour, P., & Brannon, J. (1993). The Functional Assessment of Cancer Therapy scale: Development and validation of the general measure. *Journal of Clinical Oncology, 11*(3), 570–579. https://doi.org/10.1200/JCO.1993.11.3.570

Centers for Disease Control and Prevention. (2021). *An update on cancer deaths in the United States*. https://www.cdc.gov/cancer/dcpc/research/update-on-cancer-deaths/

Chida, Y., Hamer, M., Wardle, J., & Steptoe, A. (2008). Do stress-related psychosocial factors contribute to cancer incidence and survival? *Nature Clinical Practice Oncology, 5*(8), 466–475. https://doi.org/10.1038/ncponc1134

Chochinov, H. M., Hack, T., Hassard, T., Kristjanson, L. J., McClement, S., & Harlos, M. (2005). Dignity therapy: A novel psychotherapeutic intervention for patients near the end of life. *Journal of Clinical Oncology, 23*(24), 5520–5525. https://doi.org/10.1200/JCO.2005.08.391

Cillessen, L., Johannsen, M., Speckens, A.E.M., & Zachariae, R. (2019). Mindfulness-based interventions for psychological and physical health outcomes in cancer patients and survivors: A systematic review and meta-analysis of randomized controlled trials. *Psycho-Oncology, 28*, 2257–2269. https://doi.org/10.1002/pon.5214

Cipriani, A., Barbui, C., Butler, R., Hatcher, S., & Geddes, J. (2011). Depression in adults: Drug and physical treatments. *BMJ Clinical Evidence*, 1003.

Colditz, G. A., Sellers, T. A., & Trapido, E. (2006). Epidemiology: Identifying the causes and preventability of cancer? *Nature Reviews Cancer, 6*(1), 75–83. https://doi.org/10.1038/nrc1784

Commission on Cancer. (2015). *Cancer program standards 2015: Ensuring patient-centered care*. American College of Surgeons.

Cordova, M. J., Riba, M. B., & Spiegel, D. (2017). Post-traumatic stress disorder and cancer. The Lancet. *Psychiatry, 4*(4), 330–338. https://doi.org/10.1016/S2215-0366(17)30014-7

Davidson, J. R. (2004). Remission in post-traumatic stress disorder (PTSD): Effects of sertraline as assessed by the Davidson Trauma Scale, Clinical Global Impressions and the Clinician-Administered PTSD scale. *International Clinical Psychopharmacology, 19*(2), 85–87. https://doi.org/10.1097/00004850-200403000-00005

Dempster, M., Howell, D., & McCorry, N. K. (2015). Illness perceptions and coping in physical health conditions: A meta-analysis. *Journal of Psychosomatic Research, 79*(6), 506–513. https://doi.org/10.1016/j.jpsychores.2015.10.006

Dempster, M., & McCorry, N. K. (2012). The factor structure of the revised Illness Perception Questionnaire in a population of oesophageal cancer survivors. *Psycho-Oncology, 21*(5), 524–530. https://doi.org/10.1002/pon.1927

Deshields, T. L., Howrey, H. L., & Vanderlan, J. R. (2018). Distress in oncology: Not just a psychosocial phenomenon. *Journal of Oncology Practice, 14*(12), 1800222. https://doi.org/10.1200/JOP.18.00222

Deshields, T. L., Potter, P., Olsen, S., & Liu, J. (2014). The persistence of symptom burden: Symptom experience and quality of life of cancer patients across one year. *Supportive Care in Cancer, 22*(4), 1089–1096. https://doi.org/10.1007/s00520-013-2049-3

Deshields, T., Tibbs, T., Fan, M. Y., & Taylor, M. (2006). Differences in patterns of depression after treatment for breast cancer. *Psycho-Oncology, 15*(5), 398–406. https://doi.org/10.1002/pon.962

Deshields, T., Zebrack, B., & Kennedy, V. (2013). The state of psychosocial services in cancer care in the United States. *Psycho-Oncology, 22*(3), 699–703. https://doi.org/10.1002/pon.3057

Ehde, D.M., Dillworth, T.M., & Turner, J.A., (2014). Cognitive-behavioral therapy for individuals with chronic pain. *The American Psychologist, 69*(2), 153–166. https://doi.org/10.1037/a0035747

Engel G. L. (1982). Sounding board. The biopsychosocial model and medical education. Who are to be the teachers? *The New England Journal of Medicine, 306*(13), 802–805. https://doi.org/10.1056/NEJM198204013061311

Fabrega H., Jr (1990). Psychiatric stigma in the classical and medieval period: A review of the literature. *Comprehensive psychiatry, 31*(4), 289–306. https://doi.org/10.1016/0010-440x(90)90036-r

Fann, J. R., Ell, K., & Sharpe, M. (2012). Integrating psychosocial care into cancer services. *Journal of Clinical Oncology, 30*(11), 1178–1186. https://doi.org/10.1200/JCO.2011.39.7398

Fayers, P., Bottomley, A., & EORTC Quality of Life Group, & Quality of Life Unit. (2002). Quality of life research within the EORTC-the EORTC QLQ-C30. European Organisation for Research and Treatment of Cancer. *European Journal of Cancer, 38*(Suppl 4), S125–S133. https://doi.org/10.1016/s0959-8049(01)00448-8

Fernandes, H. A., Richard, N. M., & Edelstein, K. (2019). Cognitive rehabilitation for cancer-related cognitive dysfunction: A systematic review. *Supportive Care in Cancer, 27*(9), 3253–3279. https://doi.org/10.1007/s00520-019-04866-2

Feros, D. L., Lane, L., Ciarrochi, J., & Blackledge, J. T. (2013). Acceptance and commitment therapy (ACT) for improving the lives of cancer patients: A preliminary study. *Psycho-Oncology, 22*(2), 459–464. https://doi.org/10.1002/pon.2083

Fitzgerald, P., Lo, C., Li, M., Gagliese, L., Zimmermann, C., & Rodin, G. (2015). The relationship between depression and physical symptom burden in advanced cancer. *BMJ Supportive & Palliative Care, 5*(4), 381–388. https://doi.org/10.1136/bmjspcare-2012-000380

Gale, C. K., & Millichamp, J. (2011). Generalised anxiety disorder. *BMJ Clinical Evidence*, 1002.

Getu, M.A., Chen, C., Panpan, W. Mboineki, J.F., Dhakal, I.L., & Du, R.l. (2020). The effect of cognitive behavioral therapy on the quality of life of breast cancer patients: A systematic review and meta-analysis of randomized controlled trials. *Quality of Life Research, 30*, 367–384. https://doi.org/10.1007/s11136-020-02665-5

Gibbons, A., Groarke, A., & Sweeney, K. (2016). Predicting general and cancer-related distress in women with newly diagnosed breast cancer. *BMC Cancer, 16*(1), 1–9. https://doi.org/10.1186/s12885-016-2964-z

González-Fernández, S., & Fernández-Rodríguez, C. (2019). Acceptance and commitment therapy in cancer: Review of applications and findings. *Behavioral Medicine, 45*(3), 255–269. https://doi.org/10.1080/08964289.2018.1452713

Götze, H., Brähler, E., Gansera, L., Polze, N., & Köhler, N. (2014). Psychological distress and quality of life of palliative cancer patients and their caring relatives during home care. *Supportive Care in Cancer, 22*(10), 2775–2782. https://doi.org/10.1007/s00520-014-2257-5

Grassi, L., & Riba, M. (2020). Cancer and severe mental illness: Bi-directional problems and potential solutions. *Psycho-Oncology, 29*(10), 1445–1451. https://doi.org/10.1002/pon.5534

Gupta, D., Braun, D. P., & Staren, E. D. (2012). Association between changes in quality of life scores and survival in non-small cell lung cancer patients. *European Journal of Cancer Care, 21*(5), 614–622. https://doi.org/10.1111/j.1365-2354.2012.01332.x

Hagmann, C., Cramer, A., Kestenbaum, A., Durazo, C., Downey, A., Russell, M., Geluz, J., Ma, J. D., & Roeland, E. J. (2018). Evidence-based palliative care approaches to non-pain physical symptom management in cancer patients. *Seminars in Oncology Nursing, 34*(3), 227–240. https://doi.org/10.1016/j.soncn.2018.06.004

Haller, H., Winkler, M. M., Klose, P., Dobos, G., Kuemmel, S., & Cramer, H. (2017). Mindfulness-based interventions for women with breast cancer: An updated systematic review and meta-analysis. *Acta oncologica, 56*(12), 1665–1676. https://doi.org/10.1080/0284186X.2017.1342862

Hamer, M., Chida, Y., & Molloy, G. J. (2009). Psychological distress and cancer mortality. *Journal of Psychosomatic Research, 66*(3), 255–258. https://doi.org/10.1016/j.jpsychores.2008.11.002

Hayes, S., Strosahl, K., & Wilson, K. (1999). *Acceptance and commitment therapy: An experiential approach to behavior change.* Guildford Press.

Hilfiker, R., Meichtry, A., Eicher, M., Nilsson Balfe, L., Knols, R. H., Verra, M. L., & Taeymans, J. (2018). Exercise and other non-pharmaceutical interventions for cancer-related fatigue in patients during or after cancer treatment: a systematic review incorporating an indirect-comparisons meta-analysis. *British Journal of Sports Medicine, 52*(10), 651–658. https://doi.org/10.1136/bjsports-2016-096422

Hill, J., Holcombe, C., Clark, L., Boothby, M. R., Hincks, A., Fisher, J., Tufail, S., & Salmon, P. (2011). Predictors of onset of depression and anxiety in the year after diagnosis of breast cancer. *Psychological Medicine, 41*(7), 1429–1436. https://doi.org/10.1017/S0033291710001868

Holland, J. C. (Ed.). (2010). *Psycho-oncology.* Oxford University Press. https://doi.org/10.1093/med/9780195367430.001.0001

Hulbert-Williams, N. J., Storey, L., & Wilson, K. G. (2015). Psychological interventions for patients with cancer: Psychological flexibility and the potential utility of acceptance and commitment therapy. *European Journal of Cancer Care, 24*(1), 15–27. https://doi.org/10.1111/ecc.12223

Institute of Medicine. (2013). *Delivering high-quality cancer care: Charting a new course for a system in crisis.* The National Academies Press. https://doi.org/10.17226/18359

Irwin, K. E., Park, E. R., Fields, L. E., Corveleyn, A. E., Greer, J. A., Perez, G. K., Callaway, C. A., Jacobs, J. M., Nierenberg, A. A., Temel, J. S., Ryan, D. P., & Pirl, W. F. (2019). Bridge: Person-centered collaborative care for patients with serious mental illness and cancer. *The Oncologist, 24*(7), 901–910. https://doi.org/10.1634/theoncologist.2018-0488

Jia, Y., Li, F., Liu, Y. F., Zhao, J. P., Leng, M. M., & Chen, L. (2017). Depression and cancer risk: A systematic review and meta-analysis. *Public Health, 149*, 138–148. https://doi.org/10.1016/j.puhe.2017.04.026

Johnson, J. A., Rash, J. A., Campbell, T. S., Savard, J., Gehrman, P. R., Perlis, M., Carlson, L. E., & Garland, S. N. (2016). A systematic review and meta-analysis of randomized controlled trials of cognitive behavior therapy for insomnia (CBT-I) in cancer survivors. *Sleep Medicine Reviews, 27*, 20–28. https://doi.org/10.1016/j.smrv.2015.07.001

Kastbom, L., Milberg, A., & Karlsson, M. (2017). A good death from the perspective of palliative cancer patients. *Supportive Care in Cancer, 25*, 933–939. https://doi.org/10.1007/s00520-016-3483-9

Kiecolt-Glaser, J. K., Robles, T. F., Heffner, K. L., Loving, T. J., & Glaser, R. (2002). Psychooncology and cancer: Psychoneuroimmunology and cancer. *Annals of Oncology, 13*(Suppl 4), 165–169. https://doi.org/10.1093/annonc/mdf655

Kisely, S., Crowe, E., & Lawrence, D. (2013). Cancer-related mortality in people with mental illness. *JAMA Psychiatry, 70*(2), 209–217. https://doi.org/10.1001/jamapsychiatry.2013.278

Krebber, A. M., Buffart, L. M., Kleijn, G., Riepma, I. C., de Bree, R., Leemans, C. R., Becker, A., Brug, J., van Straten, A., Cuijpers, P., & Verdonck-de Leeuw, I. M. (2014). Prevalence of depression in cancer patients: A meta-analysis of diagnostic interviews and self-report instruments. *Psycho-Oncology, 23*(2), 121–130. https://doi.org/10.1002/pon.3409

Kripke D. F. (2016). Hypnotic drug risks of mortality, infection, depression, and cancer: but lack of benefit. *F1000Research, 5*, 918. https://doi.org/10.12688/f1000research.8729.3

Kroenke, K., Spitzer, R. L., & Williams, J. B. (2001). The PHQ-9: validity of a brief depression severity measure. *Journal of General Internal Medicine, 16*(9), 606–613. https://doi.org/10.1046/j.1525-1497.2001.016009606.x

Kübler-Ross, E. (1969). *On death and dying.* Collier Books/Macmillan Publishing Co.

Langford, D. J., Cooper, B., Paul, S., Humphreys, J., Keagy, C., Conley, Y. P., Hammer, M. J., Levine, J. D., Wright, F., Melisko, M., Miaskowski, C., & Dunn, L. B. (2017). Evaluation of coping as a mediator of the relationship between stressful life events and cancer-related distress. *Health Psychology, 36*(12), 1147–1160. https://doi.org/10.1037/hea0000524

Lebel, S., Ozakinci, G., Humphris, G., Mutsaers, B., Thewes, B., Prins, J., Dinkel, A., Butow, P., & University of Ottawa Fear of Cancer Recurrence Colloquium attendees. (2016). From normal response to clinical problem: Definition and clinical features of fear of cancer recurrence. *Supportive Care in Cancer, 24*(8), 3265–3268. https://doi.org/10.1007/s00520-016-3272-5

Leventhal, H., Meyer, D., & Nerenz, D. (1980). The common sense representation of illness danger. *Contributions to Medical Psychology, 2*, 7-30.

Leventhal, H., Phillips, L. A., & Burns, E. (2016). The common-sense model of self-regulation (CSM): A dynamic framework for understanding illness self-management. *Journal of Behavioral Medicine, 39*(6), 935–946. https://doi.org/10.1007/s10865-016-9782-2

Li, M., Hales, S., & Rodin, G. (2010). Adjustment disorders. *Psycho-Oncology, 297*, 302. https://doi.org/10.1093/med/9780195367430.003.0041

Li, M., Kennedy, E. B., Byrne, N., Gérin-Lajoie, C., Katz, M. R., Keshavarz, H., Sellick, S., & Green, E. (2017). Systematic review and meta-analysis of collaborative care interventions for depression in patients with cancer. *Psycho-Oncology, 26*(5), 573–587. https://doi.org/10.1002/pon.4286

Liu, Z., Doege, D., Thong, M., & Arndt, V. (2020). The relationship between posttraumatic growth and health-related quality of life in adult cancer survivors: A systematic review. *Journal of Affective Disorders, 276*, 159–168. https://doi.org/10.1016/j.jad.2020.07.044

Liu, Z., Thong, M., Doege, D., Koch-Gallenkamp, L., Bertram, H., Eberle, A., Holleczek, B., Waldmann, A., Zeissig, S. R., Pritzkuleit, R., Brenner, H., & Arndt, V. (2021). Prevalence of benefit finding and posttraumatic growth in long-term cancer survivors:

Results from a multi-regional population-based survey in Germany. *British Journal of Cancer, 125* (6), 877–883. https://doi.org/10.1038/s41416-021-01473-z

Lotfi-Jam, K., Gough, K., Schofield, P., Aranda, S., & Jefford, M. (2019) A longitudinal study of four unique trajectories of psychological distress in cancer survivors after completing potentially curative treatment. *Acta Oncologica, 58*(5), 782–789. https://doi.org/10.1080/0284186X.2018.1562209

Lutgendorf, S. K., Sood, A. K., & Antoni, M. H. (2010). Host factors and cancer progression: biobehavioral signaling pathways and interventions. *Journal of Clinical Oncology, 28*(26), 4094–4099. https://doi.org/10.1200/JCO.2009.26.9357

Ma, Y., Hall, D. L., Ngo, L. H., Liu, Q., Bain, P. A., & Yeh, G. Y. (2021). Efficacy of cognitive behavioral therapy for insomnia in breast cancer: A meta-analysis. *Sleep Medicine Reviews, 55*, 101376. https://doi.org/10.1016/j.smrv.2020.101376

Maatouk, I., He, S., Becker, N., Hummel, M., Hemmer, S., Hillengass, M., Goldschmidt, H., Hartmann, M., Schellberg, D., Herzog, W., & Hillengass, J. (2018). Association of resilience with health-related quality of life and depression in multiple myeloma and its precursors: Results of a German cross-sectional study. *BMJ Open, 8*(7), e021376. https://doi.org/10.1136/bmjopen-2017-021376

Magai, C., Consedine, N., Neugut, A. I., & Hershman, D. L. (2007). Common psychosocial factors underlying breast cancer screening and breast cancer treatment adherence: A conceptual review and synthesis. *Journal of Women's Health (2002), 16*(1), 11–23. https://doi.org/10.1089/jwh.2006.0024

Martínez, M., Arantzamendi, M., Belar, A., Carrasco, J. M., Carvajal, A., Rullán, M., & Centeno, C. (2017). "Dignity therapy," a promising intervention in palliative care: A comprehensive systematic literature review. *Palliative Medicine, 31*(6), 492–509. https://doi.org/10.1177/0269216316665562

McFarland, D. C., Hlubocky, F., Susaimanickam, B., O'Hanlon, R., & Riba, M. (2019). Addressing depression, burnout, and suicide in oncology physicians. American Society of Clinical Oncology Educational Book. American Society of Clinical Oncology. *Annual Meeting, 39*, 590–598. https://doi.org/10.1200/EDBK_239087

Meeker, C. R., Geynisman, D. M., Egleston, B. L., Hall, M. J., Mechanic, K. Y., Bilusic, M., Plimack, E. R., Martin, L. P., von Mehren, M., Lewis, B., & Wong, Y. N. (2016). Relationships among financial distress, emotional distress, and overall distress in insured patients with cancer. *Journal of Oncology Practice, 12*(7), e755–e764. https://doi.org/10.1200/JOP.2016.011049

Mehnert, A., Brähler, E., Faller, H., Härter, M., Keller, M., Schulz, H., Wegscheider, K., Weis, J., Boehncke, A., Hund, B., Reuter, K., Richard, M., Sehner, S., Sommerfeldt, S., Szalai, C., Wittchen, H. U., & Koch, U. (2014). Four-week prevalence of mental disorders in patients with cancer across major tumor entities. *Journal of Clinical Oncology, 32*(31), 3540–3546. https://doi.org/10.1200/JCO.2014.56.0086

Mehnert, A., Hartung, T. J., Friedrich, M., Vehling, S., Brähler, E., Härter, M., Keller, M., Schulz, H., Wegscheider, K., Weis, J., Koch, U., & Faller, H. (2018). One in two cancer patients is significantly distressed: Prevalence and indicators of distress. *Psycho-Oncology, 27*(1), 75–82. https://doi.org/10.1002/pon.4464

Mitchell, A. J., Chan, M., Bhatti, H., Halton, M., Grassi, L., Johansen, C., & Meader, N. (2011). Prevalence of depression, anxiety, and adjustment disorder in oncological, haematological, and palliative-care settings: a meta-analysis of 94 interview-based studies. The Lancet. *Oncology, 12*(2), 160–174. https://doi.org/10.1016/S1470-2045(11)70002-X

Mosher, C. E., Winger, J. G., Given, B. A., Shahda, S., & Helft, P. R. (2017). A systematic review of psychosocial interventions for colorectal cancer patients. *Supportive Care in Cancer, 25*, 2349–2362. https://doi.org/10.1007/s00520-017-3693-9

Mutsaers, B., Butow, P., Dinkel, A., Humphris, G., Maheu, C., Ozakinci, G., Prins, J., Sharpe, L., Smith, A. B., Thewes, B., & Lebel, S. (2020). Identifying the key characteristics of clinical fear of cancer recurrence: An international Delphi study. *Psycho-Oncology, 29*(2), 430–436. https://doi.org/10.1002/pon.5283

Nass, S. J., Beaupin, L. K., Demark-Wahnefried, W., Fasciano, K., Ganz, P. A., Hayes-Lattin, B., Hudson, M. M., Nevidjon, B., Oeffinger, K. C., Rechis, R., Richardson, L. C., Seibel, N. L., & Smith, A. W. (2015). Identifying and addressing the needs of adolescents and young adults with cancer: summary of an Institute of Medicine workshop. *The Oncologist, 20*(2), 186–195. https://doi.org/10.1634/theoncologist.2014-0265

National Cancer Institute. (2016). *Late side effects of cancer treatment.* Author. Retrieved from https://www.cancer.gov/about-cancer/coping/survivorship/late-effects

National Comprehensive Cancer Network (NCCN). (2021). *Clinical practice guidelines in oncology: Distress management. Version 2.2021.* https://www.nccn.org/professionals/physician_gls/pdf/distress.pdf

Nielsen, S., Sabioni, P., Trigo, J. M., Ware, M. A., Betz-Stablein, B. D., Murnion, B., Lintzeris, N., Khor, K. E., Farrell, M., Smith, A., & Le Foll, B. (2017). Opioid-sparing effect of cannabinoids: A systematic review and meta-analysis. *Neuropsychopharmacology, 42*(9), 1752–1765. https://doi.org/10.1038/npp.2017.51

Nipp, R. D., Greer, J. A., El-Jawahri, A., Moran, S. M., Traeger, L., Jacobs, J. M., Jacobsen, J. C., Gallagher, E. R., Park, E. R., Ryan, D. P., Jackson, V. A., Pirl, W. F., & Temel, J. S. (2017). Coping and prognostic awareness in patients with advanced cancer. *Journal of Clinical Oncology, 35*(22), 2551–2557. https://doi.org/10.1200/JCO.2016.71.3404

Nixon, J. L., Brown, B., Pigott, A. E., Turner, J., Brown, E., Bernard, A., Wall, L. R., Ward, E. C., & Porceddu, S. V. (2019). A prospective examination of mask anxiety during radiotherapy for head and neck cancer and patient perceptions of management strategies. *Journal of Medical Radiation Sciences, 66*(3), 184–190. https://doi.org/10.1002/jmrs.346

Novack, D. H., Plumer, R., Smith, R. L., Ochitill, H., Morrow, G. R., & Bennett, J. M. (1979). Changes in physicians' attitudes toward telling the cancer patient. *JAMA, 241*(9), 897–900. https://doi.org/10.1001/jama.1979.03290350017012

Novy, D. M., & Aigner, C. J. (2014). The biopsychosocial model in cancer pain. *Current Opinion in Supportive and Palliative Care, 8*(2), 117–123. https://doi.org/10.1097/SPC.0000000000000046

Oerlemans, M. E., van den Akker, M., Schuurman, A. G., Kellen, E., & Buntinx, F. (2007). A meta-analysis on depression and subsequent cancer risk. *Clinical Practice and Epidemiology in Mental Health, 3*, 29. https://doi.org/10.1186/1745-0179-3-29

Oken, D. (1961). What to tell cancer patients. A study of medical attitudes. *JAMA, 175*, 1120–1128. https://doi.org/10.1001/jama.1961.03040130004002

Osborn, R. L., Demoncada, A. C., & Feuerstein, M. (2006). Psychosocial interventions for depression, anxiety, and quality of life in cancer survivors: Meta-analyses. *International Journal of Psychiatry in Medicine, 36*(1), 13–34. https://doi.org/10.2190/EUFN-RV1K-Y3TR-FK0L

Osório, F. L., Lima, M. P., & Chagas, M. H. (2015). Assessment and screening of panic disorder in cancer patients: Performance of the PHQ-PD. *Journal of Psychosomatic Research, 78*(1), 91–94. https://doi.org/10.1016/j.jpsychores.2014.09.001

Ostuzzi, G., Matcham, F., Dauchy, S., Barbui, C., & Hotopf, M. (2018). Antidepressants for the treatment of depression in people with cancer. *The Cochrane Database of Systematic Reviews, 4*(4), CD011006. https://doi.org/10.1002/14651858.CD011006.pub3

Özkan, M., Yıldırım, N., Dişçi, R., İlgün, A. S., Sarsenov, D., Alço, G., Aktepe, F., Kalyoncu, N., İzci, F., Selamoğlu, D., Ordu, Ç., Pilancı, K. N., Erdoğan, Z. İ., Eralp, Y., & Özmen, V. (2017). Roles of biopsychosocial factors in the development of breast cancer. *European Journal of Breast Health, 13*(4), 206–212. https://doi.org/10.5152/ejbh.2017.3519

Palmer, C. (2020). Cognition and cancer treatment. *Monitor on Psychology, 51*(2), 43–47.

Paredes, A. Z., Hyer, J. M., Tsilimigras, D. I., Palmer, E., Lustberg, M. B., Dillhoff, M. E., Cloyd, J. M., Tsung, A., Ejaz, A., Wells-Di Gregorio, S., & Pawlik, T. M. (2021). Association of pre-existing mental illness with all-cause and cancer-specific mortality among Medicare beneficiaries with pancreatic cancer. *HPB (International Hepato Pancreato Biliary Association), 23*(3), 451–458. https://doi.org/10.1016/j.hpb.2020.08.002

Park, C. L., & Folkman, S. (1997). Meaning in the context of stress and coping. *Review of General Psychology, 1*(2), 115–144.

Park, S., Sato, Y., Takita, Y., Tamura, N., Ninomiya, A., Kosugi, T., Sado, M., Nakagawa, A., Takahashi, M., Hayashida, T., & Fujisawa, D. (2020). Mindfulness-based cognitive therapy for psychological distress, fear of cancer recurrence, fatigue, spiritual well-being, and quality of life in patients with breast cancer: A randomized controlled trial. *Journal of Pain and Symptom Management, 60*(2), 381-389. https://doi.org/10.1016/j.jpainsymman.2020.02.017

Paskett, E. D., Pennell, M. L., Ruffin, M. T., Weghorst, C. M., Lu, B., Hade, E. M., Peng, J., Bernardo, B. M., & Wewers, M. E. (2020). A multi-level model to understand cervical cancer disparities in Appalachia. *Cancer Prevention Research (Philadelphia, PA), 13*(3), 223–228. https://doi.org/10.1158/1940-6207.CAPR-19-0239

Pedersen, A. F., & Zachariae, R. (2010). Cancer, acute stress disorder, and repressive coping. *Scandinavian Journal of Psychology, 51*(1), 84–91. https://doi.org/10.1111/j.1467-9450.2009.00727.x

Pikhart, H., & Pikhartova, J. (2015). *The relationship between psychosocial risk factors and health outcomes of chronic diseases: A review of the evidence for cancer and cardiovascular diseases.* WHO Regional Office for Europe. https://www.euro.who.int/en/publications/abstracts/relationship-between-psychosocial-risk-factors-and-health-outcomes-of-chronic-diseases-a-review-of-the-evidence-for-cancer-and-cardiovascular-diseases-the

Pirl, W.F., Fann, J.R., Greer, J.A., Braun, I., Deshields, T., Fulcher, C., Harvey, E., Holland, J., Kennedy, V., Lazenby, M., Wagner, L., Underhill, M., Walker, D.K., Zabora, J., Zebrack, B., & Bardwell, W.A. (2014). Recommendations for the implementation of distress screening programs in cancer centers: Report from the American Psychosocial Oncology Society (APOS), Association of Oncology Social Work (AOSW), and Oncology Nursing Society (ONS) joint task force. *Cancer, 120,* 2946-2954. https://doi.org/10.1002/cncr.28750

Popa-Velea, O., Diaconescu, L., Jidveian Popescu, M., & Truţescu, C. (2017). Resilience and active coping style: Effects on the self-reported quality of life in cancer patients. *International Journal of Psychiatry in Medicine, 52*(2), 124–136. https://doi.org/10.1177/0091217417720895

Portenoy, R. K., Thaler, H. T., Kornblith, A. B., Lepore, J. M., Friedlander-Klar, H., Kiyasu, E., Sobel, K., Coyle, N., Kemeny, N., & Norton, L. (1994). The Memorial Symptom Assessment Scale: An instrument for the evaluation of symptom prevalence, characteristics and distress. *European Journal of Cancer, 30*(9), 1326–1336. https://doi.org/10.1016/0959-8049(94)90182-1

Qaseem, A., Kansagara, D., Forciea, M. A., Cooke, M., Denberg, T. D., & Clinical Guidelines Committee of the American College of Physicians. (2016). Management of chronic insomnia disorder in adults: A clinical practice guideline from the American College of Physicians. *Annals of Internal Medicine, 165,* 125–133. https://doi.org/10.7326/M15-2175

Quinn, G. P., Sanchez, J. A., Sutton, S. K., Vadaparampil, S. T., Nguyen, G. T., Green, B. L., Kanetsky, P. A., & Schabath, M. B. (2015). Cancer and lesbian, gay, bisexual, transgender/transsexual, and queer/questioning (LGBTQ) populations. *CA: A Cancer Journal for Clinicians, 65*(5), 384–400. https://doi.org/10.3322/caac.21288

Rasmussen, V., Turnell, A., Butow, P., Juraskova, I., Kirsten, L., Wiener, L., Patenaude, A., Hoekstra-Weebers, J., Grassi, L., and on behalf of the IPOS Research Committee (2016). Burnout among psychosocial oncologists: An application and extension of the effort–reward imbalance model. *Psycho-Oncology, 25,* 194–202. https://doi.org/10.1002/pon.3902

Reiff, C. M., Richman, E. E., Nemeroff, C. B., Carpenter, L. L., Widge, A. S., Rodriguez, C. I., Kalin, N. H., McDonald, W. M., & the Work Group on Biomarkers and Novel Treatments, a Division of the American Psychiatric Association Council of Research. (2020). Psychedelics and psychedelic-assisted psychotherapy. *The American Journal of Psychiatry, 177*(5), 391–410. https://doi.org/10.1176/appi.ajp.2019.19010035

Rohde, R. L., Adjei Boakye, E., Challapalli, S. D., Patel, S. H., Geneus, C. J., Tobo, B. B., Simpson, M. C., Mohammed, K. A., Deshields, T., Varvares, M. A., & Osazuwa-Peters, N. (2018). Prevalence and sociodemographic factors associated with depression among hospitalized patients with head and neck cancer-Results from a national study. *Psycho-Oncology, 27*(12), 2809–2814. https://doi.org/10.1002/pon.4893

Romero-Sandoval, E. A., Fincham, J. E., Kolano, A. L., Sharpe, B. N., & Alvarado-Vázquez, P. A. (2018). Cannabis for chronic pain: Challenges and considerations. *Pharmacotherapy, 38*(6), 651–662. https://doi.org/10.1002/phar.2115

Rush, A. J., Trivedi, M. H., Wisniewski, S. R., Nierenberg, A. A., Stewart, J. W., Warden, D., Niederehe, G., Thase, M. E., Lavori, P. W., Lebowitz, B. D., McGrath, P. J., Rosenbaum, J. F., Sackeim, H. A., Kupfer, D. J., Luther, J., & Fava, M. (2006). Acute and longer-term outcomes in depressed outpatients requiring one or several treatment steps: a STAR*D report. *The American Journal of Psychiatry, 163*(11), 1905–1917. https://doi.org/10.1176/ajp.2006.163.11.1905

Sansom-Daly, U. M., & Wakefield, C. E. (2013). Distress and adjustment among adolescents and young adults with cancer: An empirical and conceptual review. *Translational Pediatrics, 2*(4), 167–197. https://doi.org/10.3978/j.issn.2224-4336.2013.10.06

Saracino, R. M., Rosenfeld, B., & Nelson, C. J. (2016). Towards a new conceptualization of depression in older adult cancer patients: a review of the literature. *Aging & Mental Health, 20*(12), 1230–1242. https://doi.org/10.1080/13607863.2015.1078278

Satin, J. R., Linden, W., & Phillips, M. J. (2009). Depression as a predictor of disease progression and mortality in cancer patients: A meta-analysis. *Cancer, 115*(22), 5349–5361. https://doi.org/10.1002/cncr.24561

Shand, L. K., Cowlishaw, S., Brooker, J. E., Burney, S., & Ricciardelli, L. A. (2015). Correlates of post-traumatic stress symptoms and growth in cancer patients: a systematic review and meta-analysis. *Psycho-Oncology, 24*(6), 624–634. https://doi.org/10.1002/pon.3719

Shapiro, J. P., McCue, K., Heyman, E. N., Dey, T., & Haller, H. S. (2010). Coping-related variables associated with individual differences in adjustment to cancer. *Journal of Psychosocial Oncology, 28*(1), 1–22. https://doi.org/10.1080/07347330903438883

Sharpe, M., Walker, J., Holm Hansen, C., Martin, P., Symeonides, S., Gourley, C., Wall, L., Weller, D., Murray, G., & SMaRT (Symptom Management Research Trials) Oncology-2 Team. (2014). Integrated collaborative care for comorbid major depression in patients with cancer (SMaRT Oncology-2): A multicentre randomised controlled effectiveness trial. *Lancet (London, England), 384*(9948), 1099–1108. https://doi.org/10.1016/S0140-6736(14)61231-9

Siegel, R. L., Miller, K. D., & Jemal, A. (2019). *Cancer statistics, 2019. CA: A Cancer Journal for Clinicians, 69*(1), 7–34. https://doi.org/10.3322/caac.21551

Simard, S., Thewes, B., Humphris, G., Dixon, M., Hayden, C., Mireskandari, S., & Ozakinci, G. (2013). Fear of cancer recurrence in adult cancer survivors: A systematic review of quantitative studies. *Journal of Cancer Survivorship: Research and Practice, 7*(3), 300–322. https://doi.org/10.1007/s11764-013-0272-z

Slaughter, J. R., Jain, A., Holmes, S., Reid, J. C., Bobo, W., & Sherrod, N. B. (2000). Panic disorder in hospitalized cancer patients. *Psycho-Oncology, 9*(3), 253–258. https://doi.org/10.1002/1099-1611(200005/06)9:3<253::aid-pon449>3.0.co;2-c

Slee, A., Nazareth, I., Bondaronek, P., Liu, Y., Cheng, Z., & Freemantle, N. (2019). Pharmacological treatments for generalised anxiety disorder: A systematic review and network meta-analysis. *Lancet (London, England), 393*(10173), 768–777. https://doi.org/10.1016/S0140-6736(18)31793-8

Smedslund, G., Berg, R. C., Hammerstrøm, K. T., Steiro, A., Leiknes, K. A., Dahl, H. M., & Karlsen, K. (2011). Motivational interviewing for substance abuse. *The Cochrane Database of Systematic Reviews*, (5), CD008063. https://https://doi.org/.org/10.1002/14651858.CD008063.pub2

Snaith, R. P. (2003). The Hospital Anxiety and Depression Scale. *Health and Quality of Life Outcomes, 1*, 29. https://doi.org/10.1186/1477-7525-1-29

Solmi, M., Firth, J., Miola, A., Fornaro, M., Frison, E., Fusar-Poli, P., Dragioti, E., Shin, J. I., Carvalho, A. F., Stubbs, B., Koyanagi, A., Kisely, S., & Correll, C. U. (2020). Disparities in cancer screening in people with mental illness across the world versus the general population: Prevalence and comparative meta-analysis including 4,717,839 people. The Lancet. *Psychiatry, 7*(1), 52–63. https://doi.org/10.1016/S2215-0366(19)30414-6

Spiegel, D., & Giese-Davis, J. (2003). Depression and cancer: Mechanisms and disease progression. *Biological Psychiatry, 54*(3), 269–282. https://doi.org/10.1016/s0006-3223(03)00566-3

Spitzer, R. L., Kroenke, K., Williams, J. B., & Löwe, B. (2006). A brief measure for assessing generalized anxiety disorder: The GAD-7. *Archives of Internal Medicine, 166*(10), 1092–1097. https://doi.org/10.1001/archinte.166.10.1092

Staren, E. D., Gupta, D., & Braun, D. P. (2011). The prognostic role of quality of life assessment in breast cancer. *The Breast Journal, 17*(6), 571–578. https://doi.org/10.1111/j.1524-4741.2011.01151.x

Tedeschi, R.G., & Calhoun, L.G. (2004). *Posttraumatic growth: Conceptual foundation and empirical evidence.* Erlbaum.

Teo, I., Krishnan, A., & Lee, G. L. (2019). Psychosocial interventions for advanced cancer patients: A systematic review. *Psycho-oncology, 28*(7), 1394–1407. https://doi.org/10.1002/pon.5103

Tucker, P., Zaninelli, R., Yehuda, R., Ruggiero, L., Dillingham, K., & Pitts, C. D. (2001). Paroxetine in the treatment of chronic posttraumatic stress disorder: Results of a placebo-controlled, flexible-dosage trial. *The Journal of Clinical Psychiatry, 62*(11), 860–868. https://doi.org/10.4088/jcp.v62n1105

US Cancer Statistics Working Group. (2020). *U.S. cancer statistics data visualizations tool, based on 2019 submission data (1999–2017).* US Department of Health and Human Services, Centers for Disease Control and Prevention and National Cancer Institute. https://www.cdc.gov/cancer/dataviz

Ussher, J., Kirsten, L., Butow, P., & Sandoval, M. (2006). What do cancer support groups provide which other supportive relationships do not? The experience of peer support groups for people with cancer. *Social Science & Medicine, 62*(10), 2565–2576. https://doi.org/10.1016/j.socscimed.2005.10.034

van Beek, F. E., Wijnhoven, L., Jansen, F., Custers, J., Aukema, E. J., Coupé, V., Cuijpers, P., van der Lee, M. L., Lissenberg-Witte, B. I., Wijnen, B., Prins, J. B., & Verdonck-de Leeuw, I. M. (2019). Prevalence of adjustment disorder among cancer patients, and the reach, effectiveness, cost-utility and budget impact of tailored psychological treatment: study protocol of a randomized controlled trial. *BMC Psychology, 7*(1), 89. https://doi.org/10.1186/s40359-019-0368-y

Wagner, L. I., Schink, J., Bass, M., Patel, S., Diaz, M. V., Rothrock, N., Pearman, T., Gershon, R., Penedo, F. J., Rosen, S., & Cella, D. (2015). Bringing PROMIS to practice: Brief and precise symptom screening in ambulatory cancer care. *Cancer, 121*(6), 927–934. https://doi.org/10.1002/cncr.29104

Ware, J. E., Jr, & Sherbourne, C. D. (1992). The MOS 36-item short-form health survey (SF-36). I. Conceptual framework and item selection. *Medical Care, 30*(6), 473–483.

Watts, B. V., Schnurr, P. P., Mayo, L., Young-Xu, Y., Weeks, W. B., & Friedman, M. J. (2013). Meta-analysis of the efficacy of treatments for posttraumatic stress disorder. *The Journal of Clinical Psychiatry, 74*(6), e541–e550. https://doi.org/10.4088/JCP.12r08225

Whiting, P. F., Wolff, R. F., Deshpande, S., Di Nisio, M., Duffy, S., Hernandez, A. V., Keurentjes, J. C., Lang, S., Misso, K., Ryders, S., Schmidlkofer, S., Westwood, M., & Kleijnen, J. (2015). Cannabinoids for medical use: A systematic review and meta-analysis. *JAMA, 313*(24), 2456–2473. https://doi.org/10.1001/jama.2015.6358

Willems, R. A. Bolman, C. A. W., Lechner, L., Mesters, I., Gunn, K. M., Skrabal Ross, X., & Olver, I. (2020). Online interventions aimed at reducing psychological distress in cancer patients: Evidence update and suggestions for future directions. *Current Opinion in Supportive and Palliative Care, 14*(1), 27–39. https://doi.org/10.1097/SPC.0000000000000483

Xiong, G. L., Pinkhasov, A., Mangal, J. P., Huang, H., Rado, J., Gagliardi, J., Demoss, D., Karol, D., Suo, S., Lang, M., Stern, M., Spearman, E. V., Onate, J., Annamalai, A., Saliba, Z., Heinrich, T., & Fiedorowicz, J. G. (2020). QTc monitoring in adults with medical and psychiatric comorbidities: Expert consensus from the Association of Medicine and Psychiatry. *Journal of Psychosomatic Research, 135*, 110138. https://doi.org/10.1016/j.jpsychores.2020.110138

Xunlin, N., Lau, Y., & Klainin-Yobas, P. (2020). The effectiveness of mindfulness-based interventions among cancer patients and survivors: A systematic review and meta-analysis. *Supportive Care in Cancer, 28*, 1563–1578. https://doi.org/10.1007/s00520-019-05219-9

Zigmond, A. S., & Snaith, R. P. (1983). The hospital anxiety and depression scale. *Acta psychiatrica Scandinavica, 67*(6), 361–370. https://doi.org/10.1111/j.1600-0447.1983.tb09716.x

8

Appendix: Tools and Resources

The materials reproduced on the following pages can also be downloaded free of charge from the Hogrefe website after registration.

Appendix 1: ASCO Answers: Myths & Facts About Cancer
Appendix 2: Basic Cancer Terms
Appendix 3: NCCN Distress Thermometer and Problem List
Appendix 4: Patient Screening Questions for Supportive Care

How to proceed:

1. Create a user account (or, if you have already one, please log in)

For customers from the USA, Canada, and the rest of the world:
hgf.io/login-us

For European customers:
hgf.io/login-eu

2. Download your supplementary materials

Go to **My supplementary materials** in your account dashboard and enter the code below. You will automatically be redirected to the download area, where you can access and download the supplementary materials.

Code: B-REMW8T

To make sure you have permanent direct access to all the materials, we recommend that you download them and save them on your computer.

Appendix 1: ASCO Answers: Myths & Facts About Cancer

There is a lot of information about cancer available, but some of it is misleading or wrong. Here are the facts behind some of the most common cancer myths and misconceptions. Your health care team is also a good resource if you have any questions about the accuracy of anything you hear or read.

MYTH: Cancer is contagious.

FACT: Cancer is not contagious. However, some cancers are caused by viruses and bacteria that can be spread from person to person. Certain types of the human papillomavirus (HPV) have been known to cause cervical, anal, and some kinds of head and neck cancers. Hepatitis B and hepatitis C are viruses that increase the risk of developing liver cancer. Bacteria like H. pylori can cause stomach cancer. It is important to remember that while the viruses and bacteria that cause some cancers can be spread from person to person, the cancers they cause cannot be spread from person to person.

MYTH: If you have a family history of cancer, you will get it too.

FACT: Although having a family history of cancer increases your risk of developing the disease, it is not a complete prediction of your future health. An estimated 4 out of 10 cancers can be prevented by making simple lifestyle changes, such as forming healthy eating habits, maintaining a healthy weight, exercising, limiting alcoholic beverages, practicing sun safety, and avoiding tobacco products. If you have inherited certain cancer genes that put you at high risk for cancer, your doctor may recommend surgery or medications to reduce the chance that cancer will develop.

MYTH: Cancer thrives on sugar.

FACT: There is no conclusive evidence that proves eating sugar will make cancer grow and spread more quickly. All cells in the body, both healthy cells and cancer cells, depend on sugar to grow and function. However, there is no proof that eating sugar will speed up the growth of cancer or that cutting out sugar completely will slow down its growth. This doesn't mean you should eat a high-sugar diet, though. Consuming too many calories from sugar has been linked to weight gain, obesity, and diabetes, which increase the risk of developing cancer and other health problems.

MYTH: Cancer treatment is usually worse than the disease.

FACT: Although cancer treatments, such as chemotherapy and radiation therapy, can cause unpleasant and sometimes serious side effects, recent advances have resulted in many drugs and radiation treatments that have more manageable side effects. As a result, symptoms like severe nausea and vomiting, hair loss, and tissue damage are much less common. However, managing side effects, also called supportive care or palliative care, remains an important part of cancer care. Supportive care can help a person feel more comfortable at any stage of illness. People who receive treatment for cancer and treatment to ease side effects at the same time often have less severe symptoms, better quality of life, and report that they are more satisfied with treatment.

MYTH: It is easier to remain unaware you have cancer.

FACT: You should not ignore the symptoms or signs of cancer, such as a breast lump or an abnormal-looking mole. Although the thought of having cancer is frightening, talking with your doctor and getting a diagnosis will give you the power to make informed choices and seek the best possible care. Because treatment is usually more effective during the early stages of cancer, an early diagnosis often improves a person's chance of survival.

MYTH: My attitude will have an effect on my cancer.

FACT: There is no scientific evidence that a positive attitude will prevent cancer, help people with cancer live longer, or keep cancer from coming back. However, things that promote positive thinking, such as relaxation techniques, support groups, and a support network of family and friends, may improve a person's quality of life and outlook. It is important to remember that placing such an importance on attitude may lead to unnecessary guilt and disappointment if, for reasons beyond your control, your health does not improve.

See p. 78 for instructions on how to obtain the PDF.

MYTH: Drug companies, the government, and the medical establishment are hiding a cure for cancer.

FACT: No one is withholding a cure for cancer. The fact is, there will not be a single cure for cancer. Hundreds of types of cancer exist, and they respond differently to various types of treatment. There is still much to learn, which is why clinical trials are essential for making progress in preventing, diagnosing, and treating cancer.

MYTH: If I'm not offered all of the tests, procedures, and treatments available, I am not getting the best cancer care.

FACT: Not every test, treatment, or procedure is right for every person. You and your doctor should discuss which ones will increase your chance of recovery and help you maintain the best quality of life. You should also discuss which ones could increase your risk of side effects and lead to unnecessary costs. If you decide after this discussion that you need more information before making treatment decisions, it may be helpful to seek a second opinion.

See p. 78 for instructions on how to obtain the PDF.

Appendix 2: Basic Cancer Terms

Ablation (a-BLAY-shun) is a catch-all word for removing or destroying body tissue. Doctors use different types of ablation for cancer, like drugs, heat, cold, hormones, surgery, or high-energy radio waves (called radiofrequency ablation).

Acute (a-CUTE) describes symptoms that get worse very quickly but do not last very long. Sometimes, symptoms that start as acute can stick around and last for a while. Then they become chronic (see below).

Atypical (ay-TIP-ih-cul) is a medical word for "abnormal." Doctors may use this word to describe cells or body tissues that look unusual under a microscope. They might also say your case is atypical if you do not have the usual symptoms of your type of cancer.

Benign (buh-NINE) means that a tumor is not cancerous. It does not spread to other parts of your body.

Biopsy (BYE-opp-see) is when a doctor removes a small piece of tissue from your body and sends it to a lab for testing. It's the main way to diagnose cancer. Your doctor may use a needle, scalpel, or other tool to do the biopsy.

Carcinoma (CAR-sin-OH-muh) is a cancer that starts in the lining of your organs or in your skin.

Chemotherapy (KEE-moh-THER-uh-pee) is a treatment that uses powerful drugs to kill cancer cells or to stop them from growing.

Chronic (CRAH-nik) describes a condition that lasts a long time.

Immunosuppressive (ih-MYOON-oh-suh-PRESS-iv) refers to treatments that turn down your body's immune system so it cannot fight infections as well. People who are about to get a bone marrow or organ transplant get these therapies to keep their bodies from rejecting the new tissue.

Immunotherapy (ih-MYOON-oh-THER-uh-pee) is a treatment that stimulates the immune system to help the body fight diseases like cancer.

In situ (in SIGH-too) describes cancer that has not spread to other tissue nearby.

Malignant (muh-LIG-nant) refers to cancer cells that can invade and kill nearby tissue and spread to other parts of your body.

Mass is a medical word for "lump."

Metastasis (meh-TASS-tuh-sis) is the spread of cancer from the place where it started. If it has spread far, doctors will call it "distant metastasis." The word for more than one metastasis is "metastases" (meh-TASS-tuh-sees). If the cancer has spread, your doctor may say it has "metastasized."

Oncology (on-COLL-uh-gee) is the type of medicine that focuses on cancer. Doctors who specialize in oncology are called oncologists. Other health professionals like nurses and pharmacists can specialize in oncology, too.

Primary cancer is the original cancer in your body. If the disease spreads or comes back, this is called metastasis.

Prognosis (prog-NO-sis) is a medical word for "outlook." It includes your chances of recovering from the cancer, the chances the disease will come back, and your doctor's predictions for the course of the disease. Even if you have the same type of cancer as someone else, your prognosis will be unique to you.

Radiotherapy (RAY-dee-oh-THER-uh-pee) is a treatment that uses radiation to kill cancer cells and shrink tumors. It is also called "radiation therapy." You might get it from outside the body through special machines, or your doctor might put a tiny radioactive implant inside the part of your body where the cancer is (brachytherapy).

See p. 78 for instructions on how to obtain the PDF.

Recurrence (ree-CUR-ents) means the cancer has come back after treatment. It can happen at the place where the cancer started ("local"), near where it started ("regional"), or farther away in your body ("distant").

Refractory (ree-FRACK-tor-ee) describes a condition that does not get better with treatment. Your doctor may also say your cancer is resistant.

Remission (reh-MIH-shun) means your signs and symptoms of cancer have gone away. If you have no more signs or symptoms at all, it's a full remission. If you still have some but not as many as before, it's a partial remission. Remission does not necessarily mean your cancer has been cured; it means the disease is under control.

Secondary cancer is a new primary cancer that appears after you've already been treated for cancer. This cancer is different from the one you already had.

Stage is a term doctors use to describe how far along your cancer is. The stages are 0 through IV, and the higher the number, the more advanced the disease is. The stage is based on how big the tumor is, whether your lymph nodes contain the cancer, and whether the disease has spread to other parts of your body.

Targeted therapy is a treatment that specifically identifies and targets cancer cells.

Tumor (TOO-mer) is an abnormal lump of body tissue. You can get a tumor if cells grow and copy themselves too fast or fail to die when they should. A tumor can be malignant (cancerous) or benign (not cancerous).

See p. 78 for instructions on how to obtain the PDF.

Appendix 3: NCCN Distress Thermometer and Problem List

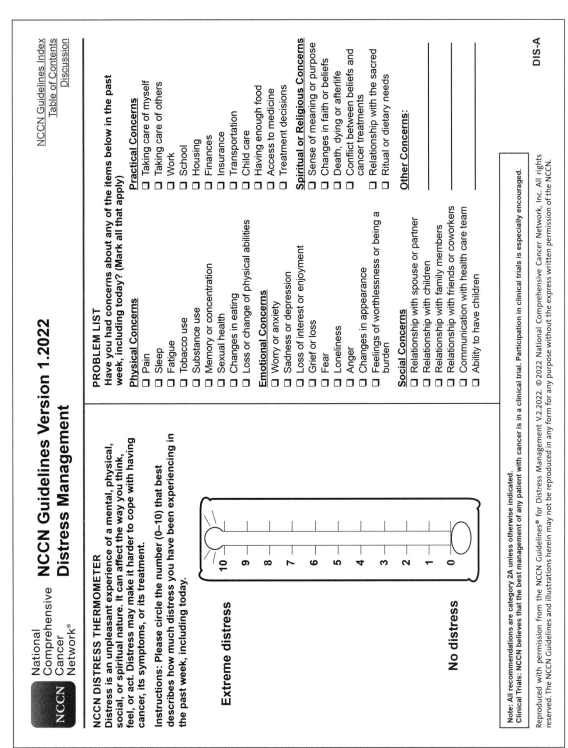

NCCN Guidelines Index
Table of Contents
Discussion

National Comprehensive Cancer Network®

NCCN Guidelines Version 1.2022

Distress Management

NCCN DISTRESS THERMOMETER

Distress is an unpleasant experience of a mental, physical, social, or spiritual nature. It can affect the way you think, feel, or act. Distress may make it harder to cope with having cancer, its symptoms, or its treatment.

Instructions: Please circle the number (0–10) that best describes how much distress you have been experiencing in the past week, including today.

Extreme distress

10
9
8
7
6
5
4
3
2
1
0

No distress

PROBLEM LIST

Have you had concerns about any of the items below in the past week, including today? (Mark all that apply)

Physical Concerns
- ❏ Pain
- ❏ Sleep
- ❏ Fatigue
- ❏ Tobacco use
- ❏ Substance use
- ❏ Memory or concentration
- ❏ Sexual health
- ❏ Changes in eating
- ❏ Loss or change of physical abilities

Emotional Concerns
- ❏ Worry or anxiety
- ❏ Sadness or depression
- ❏ Loss of interest or enjoyment
- ❏ Grief or loss
- ❏ Fear
- ❏ Loneliness
- ❏ Anger
- ❏ Changes in appearance
- ❏ Feelings of worthlessness or being a burden

Social Concerns
- ❏ Relationship with spouse or partner
- ❏ Relationship with children
- ❏ Relationship with family members
- ❏ Relationship with friends or coworkers
- ❏ Communication with health care team
- ❏ Ability to have children

Practical Concerns
- ❏ Taking care of myself
- ❏ Taking care of others
- ❏ Work
- ❏ School
- ❏ Housing
- ❏ Finances
- ❏ Insurance
- ❏ Transportation
- ❏ Child care
- ❏ Having enough food
- ❏ Access to medicine
- ❏ Treatment decisions

Spiritual or Religious Concerns
- ❏ Sense of meaning or purpose
- ❏ Changes in faith or beliefs
- ❏ Death, dying or afterlife
- ❏ Conflict between beliefs and cancer treatments
- ❏ Relationship with the sacred
- ❏ Ritual or dietary needs

Other Concerns: _____

Note: All recommendations are category 2A unless otherwise indicated.
Clinical Trials: NCCN believes that the best management of any patient with cancer is in a clinical trial. Participation in clinical trials is especially encouraged.

DIS-A

See p. 78 for instructions on how to obtain the PDF.

Appendix 4: Patient Screening Questions for Supportive Care

Questions for Your Care

All patients are asked to complete this questionnaire as part of their care.

Please take a few minutes to answer the following questions to help us better address your needs.

Do you ever need help reading hospital materials? [11]   ☐ Yes

Do you need help when filing out medical forms by yourself? [11]   ☐ Yes

Check boxes below for anything that is or has been a concern in the past 7 days, or that you may be concerned about in the future.

Side Effects, Symptoms and Other Concerns [2]

- ☐ Breathing
- ☐ Constipation
- ☐ Diarrhea
- ☐ Fevers
- ☐ Nausea or vomiting
- ☐ Sleep
- ☐ Changes in urination
- ☐ Cough
- ☐ Difficulty chewing or swallowing
- ☐ Mouth Sores
- ☐ Dry mouth
- ☐ Dental/ teeth issues
- ☐ Swollen arms or legs
- ☐ Feeling full quickly or swollen abdomen
- ☐ Appearance
- ☐ Sexual intimacy or function
- ☐ Skin dry / itchy, blister / pain
- ☐ Tingling in hands / feet
- ☐ Use of tobacco / cigarettes / vaping
- ☐ Use of medications or drugs not prescribed to you
- ☐ Difficulty concentrating
- ☐ Difficulty remembering things
- ☐ Difficulty finding the words you want to say

Pain [6]

How would you rate your pain on average?

No Pain   0 ☐   2 ☐   3 ☐   4 ☐   5 ☐   6 ☐   7 ☐   8 ☐   9 ☐   10 ☐   Worst Pain Imaginable

Nutrition Concerns [2, 3]

- ☐ Weight loss or lack of appetite
- ☐ Weight gain
- ☐ Issues with taste
- ☐ Concerns about nutrition

Ability to Do Things

To what extent are you able to carry out your everyday physical activities such as walking, climbing stairs, carrying groceries, or moving a chair? [8]

Completely	Mostly	Moderately	A little	Not at all
☐	☐	☐	☐	☐

How would you rate your fatigue on average? [7]

None	Mild	Moderate	Severe	Very severe
☐	☐	☐	☐	☐

Is someone available to help you if you need it? [10]

Never	Rarely	Sometimes	Usually	Always
☐	☐	☐	☐	☐

Falls [12]

Have you had 2 or more falls in the past 6 months?   ☐ Yes

Have you been injured by a fall that required medical attention in the last 6 months?   ☐ Yes

Do you feel unsteady when walking?   ☐ Yes

See other side to complete

See p. 78 for instructions on how to obtain the PDF.

Please answer these questions to help us address what you need.

Over the <u>last 14 days</u>, how often have you been bothered by the following problems?[1]	Not at all	Several Days	More than half the days	Nearly every day
Feeling nervous, anxious or on edge	☐	☐	☐	☐
Not being able to stop or control worrying	☐	☐	☐	☐
Little interest or pleasure in doing things	☐	☐	☐	☐
Feeling down, depressed, or hopeless	☐	☐	☐	☐

	Never	Rarely	Sometimes	Often	Always
Over the <u>last 7 days</u>, I was irritated more than people knew …	☐	☐	☐	☐	☐

Check boxes below for anything that is or has been a concern in the past 7 days, or that you are concerned about in the future.

Practical Concerns [2, 9]

- ☐ Child, adult, and / or pet care issues
- ☐ Paying for food and / or housing
- ☐ Getting to / from treatment (transportation)
- ☐ Work / school
- ☐ Health insurance or no health insurance
- ☐ Paying for medication or medical expenses
- ☐ Being able to live independently or alone

Family/Caregiver Concerns[2]

- ☐ Concerns about my children
- ☐ Concerns about my partner/caregiver/other family
- ☐ Ability to have children

Spiritual / Faith / Religious Concerns[5]

- ☐ Do you struggle with the loss of meaning and joy in your life?
- ☐ Do you have religious or spiritual struggles?

Treatment or Care Concerns [4]

- ☐ I want to better understand my cancer diagnosis or stage.
- ☐ I want to better understand my prognosis or long-term outcome.
- ☐ I have concerns or questions about my treatment options, medication or my plan of care.
- ☐ I need assistance in completing a POA HC (Power of Attorney for Health Care) that allows me to select someone I trust to make medical decisions for me when I am unable to speak for myself.
- ☐ I want to talk with someone about documenting what medical treatments I would, or would not, want to receive if I were approaching the end of my life. (POLST – Practitioner Orders for Life-Sustaining Treatment)

What Matters to You

	Not at all	Not Much	Somewhat	Very Much
Continuing to work at your job or attend school	☐	☐	☐	☐
Knowing the time commitment of your treatment	☐	☐	☐	☐
Doing your hobbies/exercise activities	☐	☐	☐	☐
Maintaining your household responsibilities	☐	☐	☐	☐

Dates of upcoming special events or vacations:

Other problems or concerns [2]:

*This tool is adapted from: (1) the PHQ-4 developed by Drs. Robert L. Spitzer, Janet B.W. Wiliams, Kurt Kroenke and colleagues; (2) The National Comprehensive Cancer Network, NCCN Guidelines version 2.2018 Distress Management; (3) Kaiser, M.J., et al., Validation of the Mini Nutritional Assessment short-form (MNA-SF): a practical tool for identification of nutritional status. J Nutr Health Aging, 2009. 13(9): p. 782-8.; (4) Living Well Cancer Resource Center Distress Tool. (5) King, S. D. W., et al. (2017). Determining best methods to screen for religious/spiritual distress. Support Care Cancer (2017) 25:471–479. (6) PROMIS Item Bank v1.0 Pain Intensity Short Form 3a; (7) PROMIS Item Bank v1.0 Fatigue Short Form 4a; (8) PROMIS Item Bank v1.0 Physical Function Short Form 4a; and PROMIS item bank. (9) Live Well At Home Rapid Screen©. (10) PROMIS Item Bank Instrumental Support – Short Form 4a. (11) Cornett, S., (Sept. 30, 2009) "Assessing and Addressing Health Literacy" OJIN: The Online Journal of Issues in Nursing Vol. 14, No. 3, Manuscript 2. (12) Phelan, E. A., Mahoney, J. E., Voit, J. C., & Stevens, J. A. (2015). Assessment and Management of Fall Risk in Primary Care Settings. The Medical Clinics of North America, 99(2), 281–293. http://doi.org/10.1016/j.mcna.2014.11.004

There are no warranties of any kind whatsoever regarding the content, use, or application and disclaim any responsibility for its application or use in any form. The development of the original tool originated through a collective collaborative effort of clinicians and patient advocacies supported by the Coleman Foundation, a philanthropic, grantmaking organization.

Office Use Only:

Pt alone ☐

Pt with family ☐

Pt w/ clinician/staff ☐

v.031.02162022

See p. 78 for instructions on how to obtain the PDF.

Peer Commentaries

This is an extremely comprehensive, evidence-based, yet deeply clinical and practical book that is a must-read for any professional who is committed to helping cancer patients and their caregivers. The authors couple their profound knowledge of the current science with clinical acumen that makes the material come alive and practical. I strongly recommend this book to both trainees and advanced practitioners who want to have the most recent advances in the field at their fingertips.

Matthew Loscalzo, LCSW, APOS Fellow, Executive Director, People & Enterprise Transformation; Emeritus Professor of Supportive Care Medicine and Professor of Population Sciences at City of Hope, CA

This is an incredible resource for all psychosocial clinicians who support patients with cancer throughout their treatment trajectory and into survivor-ship. The chapter on psychological approaches to cancer care is concise and comprehensive in covering evidence-based interventions. It is essential reading for clinicians in any stage of their career.

Krista Nelson, LCSW, OSW-C, FAOSW, FAPOS, Immediate Past President, Association of Community Cancer Centers; Program Manager, Providence Cancer Institute, Portland, OR

This book provides a thorough and approachable overview of the etiology, differential diagnosis, and treatment of cancer-related anxiety and mood disorders. It is a valuable reference point for oncologists as well as psycho-social oncologists and especially useful to general mental health professionals, trainees, and medical practitioners in primary care and other noncancer specialties.

Alan Valentine, MD, FAPOS, Chair, Department of Psychiatry, The University of Texas MD Anderson Cancer Center, Houston, TX

This is a go-to resource for clinicians and trainees seeking to provide state-of-the-art, evidence-based supportive care for patients and families affected by cancer. The authors deserve high praise for not only describing the key theoretical underpinnings of the psychosocial effects of cancer but also offering practical guidance on assessing and treating the most common forms of distress experienced by this vulnerable population. The work is comprehensive yet concise and immensely informative!

Joseph A. Greer, PhD, Associate Professor of Psychology, Harvard Medical School; Co-Director, Cancer Outcomes Research & Education Program, Massachusetts General Hospital Cancer Center, Boston, MA

This book helps therapists to quickly gain understanding of the most common issues encountered with individuals impacted by cancer and to incorporate evidence-based approaches into their treatment. It is one of those go-to books you want on your bookshelf.

William Pirl, MD, MPH, Vice Chair for Psychosocial Oncology, Department of Psychosocial Oncology and Palliative Care, Dana-Farber Cancer Institute, Harvard Medical School, Boston, MA

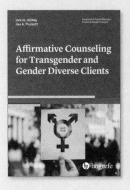
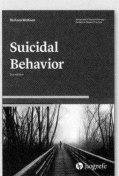
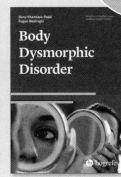
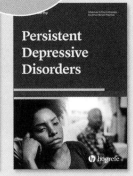
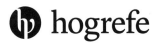

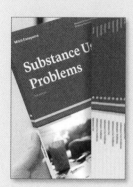
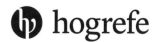